Current Topics in Microbiology
89 and Immunology

Edited by

W. Arber, Basle · S. Falkow, Seattle · W. Henle, Philadelphia
P.H. Hofschneider, Martinsried · J.H. Humphrey, London
J. Klein, Tübingen · P. Koldovský, Düsseldorf · H. Koprowski,
Philadelphia · O. Maaløe, Copenhagen · F. Melchers, Basle
R. Rott, Gießen · H.G. Schweiger, Ladenburg/Heidelberg
L. Syruček, Prague · P.K. Vogt, Los Angeles

David W. Weiss

Tumor Antigenicity and Approaches to Tumor Immunotherapy

An Outline

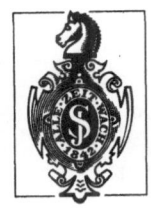

Springer-Verlag
Berlin Heidelberg New York 1980

David W. Weiss
Lautenberg Center for General and Tumor Immunology
Hebrew University – Hadassah Medical School
Jerusalem, Israel

ISBN-13:978-3-642-67499-0   e-ISBN-13:978-3-642-67497-6
DOI:10.1007/978-3-642-67497-6

Library of Congress Catalog Card Number 15-12910.

Typesetting: Fotosatz Service Weihrauch, Würzburg
2121/3321-543210

It is forbidden to despair
Nachman of Bratzlav

Contents

Introduction

This volume is not intended as review of the large literature on tumor antigenicity and efforts at tumor immunotherapy. Its purpose, rather, is to present discursively an outline of the likely approaches to immunological intervention in neoplastic diseases which present themselves today, in light of the probable antigenic properties of cancer cells. References are cited only selectively, in illustration of some of the major considerations to which allusion is made and of some of the supportive evidence. No attempt is made at inclusiveness in the citation of concepts and findings. If undue emphasis appears to be given to some aspects of the literature and only sparse documentation to others, the grounds do not lie necessarily with a critical estimation of the extent or quality of reported work, but rather with the bias of the writer who considers stress on some facets of the field more appropriate than on others for elaboration of his arguments. The references brought in support of a given point are often intentionally varied, including both reports of original work and reviews, very recent observations and contributions that gave initial impetus to investigations, in an attempt to exemplify the pertinent literature; and reference is made both to data presented and to concepts advanced. The accent placed on studies conducted by the writer and his present and former associates is motivated not by any attribution of exaggerated significance to this work, but rather by an intimacy of familiarity and by the consideration that our own efforts in the field over the past two decades have been representative of many of its fluctuating developments.

1 Tumor-Associated Antigenicity and Host Responsiveness: Basic Questions and Considerations

The central hypothesis underlying all attempts at immunological intervention in neoplastic diseases is today in danger of falling. The expectations rife only a few years ago that most, if not all, neoplasms would be found to express immunogenic determinants characteristic of the transformation event, or of the neoplastic condition per se, have come to be viewed by many investigators as the hopeful but probably unwarranted extrapolations of findings with a limited spectrum of experimental tumors in laboratory rodents [164, 213, 217, 218, 292, 424, 430], test models of very questionable relevance to neoplasia in nature [164, 425, 428].

Although there is now developing a body of more carefully adduced evidence for the distinctive antigenic properties of some spontaneously arising growths of man as well as of laboratory animals [13, 39, 65, 116, 136, 137, 158, 242, 278, 279, 336, 337, 402, 403], in addition to those of experimental neoplasms [88, 274, 443], past failures to establish the specificity of immunological responses directed against cancer cells leave standing the question whether neoplasm-unique anitgenicity is a universal, or even common, manifestation of spontaneously transformed cells. Still greater doubt has been cast on the capability of any distinguishing tumor antigens to evoke *protective* immunological reactions by the host. At least some spontaneous cancers of mice and rats do not present antigens which readily elicit protective immunity [164, 165], and even tumors experimentally induced by powerful carcinogens do not perforce possess such constituents [15, 16].

It is necessary, moreover, to hold in abeyance the surmise of a qualitative tumor-*specific* antigenicity (TSA) even with regard to neoplasms which do appear to display peculiar antigenic attributes. The biological nature and immunological behavior of antigens particularly associated with the neoplastic state remain very uncertain. Where such antigens are presumably demonstrated, they have often been discovered to be entities exhibited as well on normal cells, but primarily early in life ("fetal" or "embryonic" antigens), perhaps fleetingly and in minute quantities; or only in other tissues, sometimes highly specialized ("organ-specific" antigens); or in cells of the same type but there in categorically smaller amounts or different molecular configurations [6, 18, 19, 35, 54, 77, 138, 226, 238, 241, 253, 307, 351, 391, 223]. It is virtually impossible, accordingly, to disprove the eventuality that a seeming TSA is not, in fact, such a normal, "displacement" antigen. Even where the occurrence of such markers on normal cells is minimal, dissimilar, only transient, or restricted to specialized, perhaps immunologically sequestered, tissues, their representation (within the lifetime of the organism) among normal self-structures consigns them to a category other than that of any hypothetical antigens wholly unique to the circumstances of neoplasia, and places large constraints on their operative immunogenicity. Tumor-*associated* antigen (TAA) thus appears a far more appropriate term than tumor-specific antigen [35].

It must be said at once, however, that the decisive question to be asked from the perspective of immunological intervention in malignant disease is not whether spontaneous tumors are, on the whole, de facto immunogenic as they exist in nature, but rather whether they are *potentially* immunogenic. A clear differentiation must be made between antigenicity and immunogenicity. In the context of tumor immunology, we may define as antigen any structure of a neoplastic cell variant which is sufficiently different in kind, organization, or amount from the composition of analogous normal cells to be capable of inciting an immunological response *under appropriate conditions*. The designation "distinctive tumor antigenicity" should thus imply no more than the *potential* for immunological reactivity, or potential immunogenicity. The term immunogen, in contrast, should be restricted to tumor cell constituents whose potential immunological reactivity is realized, which by reason of their characteristics and of the suitability of host and environment actively evoke immunological responses.

Many factors impinge on the realization of immunogenic potential. In addition to the alterations in cell structure which accompany or follow neoplastic transformation, they include host genotype, age, sex, and previous experience with related antigens; external environmental variables which influence host immunological capacity; and the tissue environment in which the initial and subsequent confrontations between host and neoplastic parasite take place [423]. Some of these determinants are labile and inherently variable, and instead of static descriptions of tumor cell immunogenicity there are demanded definitions formulated precisely as a function of time and flux in the course of given host–tumor associations. This is borne out by the consideration that the amount of antigen presented [98, 161] as well as the method and route of presentation and its persistence in host tissues can cetermine whether TAAs reach the threshold of immunogenicity, quantitatively [161].

The range of factors which actuate the translation of antigenicity to immunogenicity can be extended by the investigator. Spontaneous alterations in the molecular constituents and arrangements of a tumor cell may be too small to bring the cell to the threshold of immunogenicity in a host of ordinary immunological ability. Artificial modification of TAAs can, however, bring about host responses which will be directed ultimately at the unmodified structure as well; and, nonspecific potentiation and modulation of the immunological apparatus can make for responsiveness of which the unstimulated organism is incapable. Such manipulations of antigen and host must be included within an operative perspective of the potentials of immunological reactivity toward tumor cell components.

Autoimmune reactions directed at normal cells are a not uncommon event, moreover, and evidence has been brought forward for the constant presence among the immunocyte complement in healthy subjects of clones programmed against ordinary self-components, prevented from exerting cytotoxic effects in vivo only by circulating blocking substances and perhaps also by suppressor cells [80, 371]. The proclivity for autochthonous recognition of some or many of the components of normal tissue may thus be, in fact, a pedestrian immunological reality, whith only the final cytotoxic consequences being the exceptional, pathological happening. The argument is further advanced by the proposition that the cytotoxic T lymphocyte receptor repertoire is basically directed at variants of autologous major histocompatibility complex (MHC) products [58, 140], a possibility supported by the finding that a large proportion of cytotoxic T cell precursors are programmed against such antigens [38]. Persuasive evidence that at least some TAAs may be closely related to normal MHC-coded structures has been advanced by some investigators, although the conclusion is questioned by others [64, 68, 117, 222, 257, 287, 453].

Although immunological reactivity against fetal, organ-specific, and other normal-cell antigens is likely to be compromised within the framework of self-tolerance, a degree of cognizance of tumor cells as "alien" because of the exposure of such markers at a deviant time or place or in variant amounts and arrangement is not, accordingly, improbable. Sensitization against normally occurring self-markers may result from in situ recognition of their aberrant expression by relevant lymphoid centers, as well as from systemic responsiveness to changes in antigen makeup and presentation that accompany abnormal tissue growth and damage. It is known that organ-specific antigens can be reacted to as markedly alien when they are transposed to distal body compartments, especially where the transposition is from or to sites not normally in full systemic immunological communication within the organism. Adult capacity to react toward antigens which characterize structures in early development, then eclipse, and are reintroduced experimentally in maturity has indeed been demonstrated in models not pertaining to neoplasia [389]. "Fetal" or "embryonic" antigens may persist on certain normal cells (stem cells?) throughout life, albeit at very low levels, and could in fact thereby reinforce a measure of immunological awareness of their presence, albeit normally suppressed and quiescent. Despite the tendency of some investigators to the contrary, one cannot discount the possibility that some fetal antigens on tumor cells can incite and be the targets of cytotoxic immunological reactions [18, 19, 253].

It would thus seem that host responsiveness to neoplastic cells is not conditioned wholly on their presentation of truly unique antigens, and that it may suffice if our immunotherapeutic intentions center on the detection and maneuverability of antigens merely *associated* with the neoplastic state – antigens that may be deviant from normal only in ontogeny, steric configuration, quantity, or tissue localization.

A generally assumed qualification has been that the TAAs of interest in host defensive responses are those located on the cell surface, there providing targets for immune attack, i.e., tumor-associated transplantation antigens (TATAs). This view may be an unnecessarily restricted one, however. Recent experiments conducted by *J. Vaage* (1978, personal communication; 398), suggest that immunological reactions expressed against some tumors may be manifested by a process of walling off and necrosis of the neoplastic focus akin to tubercle formation [306], rather than by direct cytotoxicity against the living transformed cells; as has also been suggested by other workers (*G.J. Svet-Moldavsky* 1978, personal communication; 459), nonlymphoid cells of stromal origin may play a large role in attracting other cell types to participate in such indirect attack or serve themselves as "natural killers." Although these findings are preliminary, they point to the possibility that TAAs other than those located on the cell surface may be involved in the elicitation of host defenses, by triggering a sequence of responses leading to tumor destruction mechanically and by change in the local tissue environment.

We can then rephrase our central question, operatively: Are the molecular changes which characterize tumor cells sufficient in themselves to allow for host immunological responsiveness, or do they at least provide a handle for extrinsic activation to immunogenictiy and host reactivity?

Host–tumor interactions in which immunological reactivity to the neoplastic variants does develop, naturally or in consequence of extrinsic intervention, present a second key question: Do the immunological mechanisms brought into play lead to inhibition or destruction of the tumor cells, are they without appreciable import for tumor cell growth, or do they cause tumor growth stimulation, directly [293, 294] or by affording protection against other, damaging facets of the response? This question, too, must be posed of each individual neoplastic process, repeatedly in the course of its evolution; and the likelihood must be entertained that the multifaceted immunological responses to antigenic stimulation have varied, changeable, and mixed implications for the fate of tumor cells [118, 451]. Even where cellular immune responses are of defensive value, distinct immunocyte populations may be responsible for cytotoxic and for cytostatic action [1, 356]. Conversely, the possibility cannot be excluded that a host cell characterized in given tests to have reactivity of given import may also have other, even contradictory, capacities, that come to light by other appropriate measurements. It is not inconceivable that the same cell can execute, under different circumstances or even simultaneously, cytotoxic, suppressor, and stromal functions toward the same or another tumor (63, 459, E.M. Fenyö 1979, personal communication; F. Vánky 1979, personal communication). This eventuality is not ruled out by findings of different surface markers on immunocytes showing distinct behavior in defined test systems; lymphoreticular cells may be flexible in the phenotypic expression of membrane determinants, which may come to the fore differentially as the cell experiences changing physiological conditions and excitation.

A third core question to which answers must be sought as basis for the construction of rational pathways to immunotherapy is addressed to tumor escape from immunological control, and to idiosyncratic host immune failure. Where tumor antigenicity, host genotype, and both external and internal environmental variables are such as to permit the mounting of tumor inhibitory immunological responses, what are the means by which clones of neoplastic cells can avoid or abort immunological attack, and what are the epigenetic circumstances that can produce precipitous host failure at effective responsiveness, systemically or in the immediate vicinity of the tumor? The earlier conception of host immunological dyscrasia and tumor "sneaking through" as primary causes for progressive neoplastic disease is no longer given prominence by many investigators; inadequate immunogenicity of those tumors that constitute the clinical problem is deemed an adequate reason for their occurrence. This view seems insufficient, however. Both direct and indirect evidence for immunological capacity of at least some organisms against at least some spontaneous neoplasms is accumulating; phenotypic immunodeficiency does appear to contribute to host susceptiviliy in certain cases, although the contribution may not be cardinal [228, 281, 282, 283, 347, 366, 368]; and numerous avenues of possible tumor cell escape from immune attack have been shown, albeit many in artifactual test systems [178, 195, 212, 215, 218]. The contributory roles to progressive neoplastic disease of host failure and tumor cell circumvention must be weighed, even though our attention now centers on the immunogenic paucity of TATAs; and the opportunities for prevention or reversal of individual host deficiency and of tumor cell evasion can be explored only against a background of comprehension of the vagaries of host and tumor cell conduct and interaction [423].

It is self-evident that the development of effectively inhibitory, escape-route-sealed immunological responses against tumor cells that have initiated progressive growth in an organism is very much more the exception than the rule in the natural history of neoplastic diseases. Can we then attain sufficient mastery over the immunological interplay, actual and potential, between tumor cells and host immunocytes to magnify and direct immune reactivity toward definitive therapeutic ends?

Much of what has been essayed so far has been an approach of trial and error, with error and only marginal success, at best, the prominent features [377, 378]. The aura of crisis which permeates the attitude to treatment of malignancies has made acceptable the introduction of immunotherapeutic procedures with only scanty foundations of rationality and laboratory experience. Many of the immunotherapeutic agents employed until now have been taken to clinical trial peremptorily, with threadbare foreknowledge of the range, conditions, and modes of their hoped-for activities. The philosophy of their use has often been based on that of other treatment modalities, and not infrequently in frontal defiance of recognized immunological principles. Thus, for instance, design of dosage and schedule of treatment with nonspecific immunomodulators has commonly ignored patent hazards of suppressor cell activation and of other eventualities of tolerance induction, as well as of the nullifying of immunological stimulation by inappropriately spaced chemo- and radiation therapy [426, 428].

It must be admitted, on the other hand, that the plight of many cancer patients gives grounds for the grasping at straws and for leaps from drawing board to clinic that would be condemned as wild acrobatics in many other areas of medicine. Moreover, the intimations of some success with immunotherapeutic intervention that have come from several programs of investigation [176, 378], albeit still tentative and limited, provide some reason to believe that further exploration is warranted. Future investigations in the clinic must be predicated, however, on a much broadened understanding of the immunology of neoplasia, and on full appreciation of the individuality and fluidity of host–tumor relationships.

The brief survey of tumor antigenicity in the light of etiology here presented is proposed as a point of departure for the examination of several major directions of immunotherapeutic attempts, currently and in the immediate future.

2 Tumor Etiology and Antigenicity

2.1 Tumors Known to be Induced by Viruses

Several distinct classes of antigens can appear on tumor cells in outcome of the presence and activities of oncogenic viruses: components of the virion itself; structures made under the genetic control of the viral genome; structures for which the host cell carries the genetic coding, with the virus acting to derepress repressed information; and configurations appearing as secondary manifestations of the disturbances taking place in the morphology and physiology of a virally infected cell [23, 59, 90, 173, 188, 307, 342].

Virus-dependent antigens may be group-specific for the agent, and may appear in common on tumors induced in different hosts [408]; they may also have degrees of specificity associated with the particular host in which the virus induced transformation, and perhaps even with individual tumors [409, 410]. Some passenger viruses infecting neoplastic cells can probably give rise to a similar diversity of antigens [222].

Although the focus of our discussion on the antigenicity of virus-induced neoplasms and of tumors secondarily infected with viruses is here on structures attending the presence and functions of the agents, it must be noted that a variety of other TAAs – fetal, organ-specific, perhaps even TSTA – may also occur on such tumors, in some instances specific for individual growths, and may compete for full expression with those directly associated with the virus [392, 400, 418, 443]. It would be erroneous, therefore, to make automatic and limited assumptions as to the range of antigens borne by neoplastic cells of viral etiology or viral superinfection; it could indeed be that antigenic markers of particular interest as resistance-inducing antigens are at times concomitants of the transformed state per se, not directly of its origin.

Similarly, there is indication that TAAs may also compete for expression on the cell surface with normal histocompatibility antigens [76, 216, 307, 367]. Such competition can bring about dilution of relevant tumor target epitopes. It may also be of interest with view to the concept that cellular immunological responsiveness is derivative of, and to an extent circumscribed by, recognition of normal self-MHC antigens [58], and that reactivity to tumor-associated membrane configurations can be affected by the arrangement of MHC locus products with other determinants [334, 456]. Clark et al. have suggested that "the particular arrangement of specific tumor antigen, organ-specific antigen, HL-A (or H-2) antigen and nonantigenic glycoprotein present on tumor membranes and in sera within a single molecular entity may explain the apparent nonimmunogenicity of metastasizing tumors . . ." [76A].

The active immunogenicity of virus-dependent antigens on tumor cells is problematic, and perhaps especially their elicitation of cytotoxic responses in the tumor host. Where the agents are transmitted vertically, or infect horizontally soon after birth, or enter the organism repeatedly in adulthood, reaction to the virus-associated antigens can lead readily to prolonged specific (partial) tolerance [90, 91, 234, 235]. This is most probable where such antigens appear early in ontogeny, expressed on infected cells for long periods prior to their final neoplastic transformation; it may also be the case where oncogenic virus infection occurs later in life and the associated antigens appear and are maintained on still-normal cells for some time preceding frank neoplasia. It could be argued indeed that the development of such tolerance is an evolutionary necessity, to facilitate survival of the organism into reproductive maturity. This consideration applies as well to immunological deportment vis-à-vis fetal and tissue-specific antigens, translocated in time and tissue geography with the neoplastic condition and expressed exaggeratedly on cells whose transformation was precipitated by different oncogenic stimuli. "Negative" acknowledgment by the immunological mechanism of such determinants, i.e., specific immunological unresponsiveness, may be a fundamental requisite of self-acceptance, alternative or in addition to a steering of active responsiveness in directions innocuous of cytotoxic consequences.

In addition, some viruses, oncogenic and incidental, can suppress immunological ability broadly [46, 168, 366]. Moreover, the mutability of many viral agents can lead to the generation of different antigens on cells transformed by the same family of viruses, with successive clonal variability even in a given neoplastic event, and thereby with resultant impediment to the development of effective acquired immunity in the course of neoplastic progression.

Certain ubiquitous oncogenic viruses pose a serious threat to survival of host populations in nature [217, 218]. Where this is the case, existing host species may indeed have evolved, for all these difficulties, highly effective immune surveillance mechanisms directed at virus dependent antigens, mechanisms perhaps already operative vis-à-vis preneoplastic cell variants. Multiple lines of immune defense may well have arisen to guarantee protection against such tumors. These neoplastic diseases may take place only in organisms whose immunological capacity has not yet matured or has been severely injured; polyoma tumors of mice are a classic example of neoplasms induced by a virus which occur naturally only in animals incapable of normal immunological reactivity [144, 217].

It may be argued, then, that many species, including man, would be subject to a very high incidence of virus-induced neoplastic disease, were it not for effective immune surveillance. Although certainly of theoretical interest, this argument does not address itself directly to the problem of those neoplastic diseases of viral, or other, etiology which *are* prevalent today in man and in animals, i.e., those tumors against which selective processes for immunological, or other, mechanisms of resistance have not (yet) developed to categorical efficacy. Nonetheless, analysis of the modes of resistance which in normal organisms prevent forms of progressive neoplasia that are prominent in immunologically impoverished ones may pave the way to immunotherapeutic (and perhaps also immunoprophylactic) intervention designed to replicate evolutionarily successful immune defenses.

In some oncogen–host relationships in nature, the evolution of host resistance appears to have been only partially effective so far, some members of a species being incapable of offering decisive opposition to oncogenesis or progressive neoplastic growth, others able to stand up to the challenge. Feline leukemia and Burkitt's lymphoma of man may be cases in point [213, 218], and it may well be that other tumors, too, including some that are rather common in populations at their present stage in phylogeny, constitute the exceptions to a generally accomplished evolution of host refractoriness. The differential virulence of different types of neoplasms may also be related in part to the relative success of ongoing selective pressures for defense. It would not seem unreasonable to hope that insight into the circumscribed and imperfect defense reactions of tumor hosts in the field, including the cancer patient, could lead to a focusing of immunotherapeutic efforts toward strengthening those safeguards which are evolving in nature but which are still incomplete or breachable.

Laboratory investigations into virus-induced neoplasia have been confined largely to tumors occurring with a high incidence in inbred animals, in many instances inbred at multiple genetic loci making for prevalence of tumors with a viral etiology. Leukemia in AKR mice is a prototype example [217]; mammary carcinomas in mice carrying the mammary tumor viruses (MTV and NIV) another [417]. Studies in outbred animals have usually been with viral variants selected for high tumorigenic potential, and propagated under artificial laboratory conditions. It is doubtful whether such models of neoplasia, including tumors appearing "spontaneously" in inbred subjects infected with oncogenic agents, bear much relevance to neoplastic disease of viral origin in nature. Selection for viral oncogenic potency and host susceptibility (or resistance), the probability that isogenicity between long-transplanted tumors and current test animals is often incomplete [412], and the relative facility of immunological manipulation in genetically homogeneous organisms remove most of the test systems employed from the realities of neoplasia in clinic and field.

Nonetheless, the wealth of data which has come from laboratory investigations of viral neoplasia cannot be disregarded as devoid of all illustrative value for the advancement of immunotherapy. It *is* of importance that cancer cure and prevention can be effected by immunological means in test systems where native host resistance is, in fact, low and where oncogenic agents or tumor isografts produce rapidly fatal disease in control animals. It is of no less interest that some degree of antitumor immunological and resistance reactivity can be demonstrated even where neoplastic disease is triggered by viruses under conditions strongly favoring immunological unresponsiveness to virus-associated antigens [10, 44, 45, 167, 367, 375, 376, 399, 416, 434].

Elucidation of the immunological interactions between experimental hosts and tumors also provides guidelines, for all the artifactuality of the models, to analysis of host-tumor equilibria in nature. To cite only one instance, recent studies in our laboratories with Rous sarcomas have revealed a consistent autochthonous preference of tumor cell recognition by murine and avian hosts despite the dominant expression of shared group-specific viral antigenicities on the transformed cells [409, 410]; this indicates that even against a background of immunological reactions manifested against antigens directly associated with an oncogenic virus, the host can mount responses distinct for the neoplasm that poses the individual challenge. Cognizance of this phenomenon in the laboratory now prescribes a search for its occurrence, and therapeutic exploitation, in human cancer. Encouragement for this search is provided by the possibility that some TATAs appearing on neoplasms under the influence of oncogenic viruses may be compound structures composed of virion- or virus-dependent and normal host cell membrane constituents [230, 325]. Such TATAs are likely to bear a considerable degree of host-associated as well as of agent-associated specificity. Evidence is also developing for the view that some virus-associated TATAs may be polymolecular entities composed of virion constituents and virus-coded products [196]. The creation of constellations of histocompatibility, virion and virus linked, and individual tumor associated antigens may well favor immunological recognition and responsiveness [58, 334, 456, 457], and facilitate "autochthonous preference"; it might also prevent the induction of specific immunological unresponsiveness, to markers determined exclusively by the presence or activities of the agent.

At the present, viral agents are incriminated clearly in the etiology of only a few types of human neoplasia. It is not out of the question, however, that further investigation will implicate viruses more widely in the causation of human tumors [5A, 168, 256]. Efforts at heightening immunity to malignant diseases of man would be buoyed, in that event, by the analogy of successful immunological intervention in many virus-initiated neoplasms of animals.

2.2 Tumors Known to be Induced by Chemical Agents and by Other Carcinogenic Stimuli

The transplantation immunogenicity of tumors produced experimentally with a variety of carcinogenic chemicals, irradiation, hormones, and certain physical irritants varies from pronounced to marginal or nonexistent, and where antigenicity is apparent, variable degrees of uniqueness associated with individual tumors, histological type, and carcinogenic stimulus have been noted [15, 147, 211, 219, 229, 290, 341, 435].

The antigens fall into different categories. Fetal, organ-associated, and other determinants not appearing in similar amounts on analogous normal cells have been detected [15, 351]. Some carcinogenic agents may activate latent, or masked, viruses either with oncogenic activity or capable of superinfection, and the TAAs of tumors so initiated or infected may include the spectrum of virus-related entities. Some antigens may reflect the consequences of other morphologic alterations, causal or incidental of the neoplastic condition, which are effected by the carcinogenic stimulus on target cells. As with virus-induced neoplasms, the TAAs of tumors produced by chemical and physical agents are often expressed to different extents by similar growths, and perhaps even by subpopulations of transformed cells originating from the same primary neoplasm; and the phenotypic expression of some TAAs can be, like that of normal histocompatibility antigens [238], an expendable concomitant of the neoplastic state, to a variable extent for different tumors [76, 210, 214].

Recent studies in our laboratories support the findings of others that strong antitumor reactivity can be manifested by immunocytes derived even from hosts with large tumor burdens [264], although, as has been the common experience of investigators, with uncertain and wavering lines of specificity. (It is apparent, moreover, that the presence of a first tumor can have important regulatory effects on concomitant immunity: removal of a primary growth is sometimes followed shortly by explosive metastatic involvement, and the suggestion has been offered, in line with not infrequent clinical observation, that "surgical excision of a tumor may not be, in all instances, in the long-term interest of the tumor-bearing host" [118].) Current experiments by our group also reemphasize the variability of immunological responses often evoked against the same tumor by different means of contact – neoplasms implanted and remaining in situ; ligation of a limb bearing the implant; surgical extirpation of the growth – and the variability of heightened responsiveness as assessed by different assays [449]. Attention is clearly mandatory to the totality of a tumor process, however initiated, and to the methodology of sensitization and testing, if an accurate picture of the immunological facets of the interaction is to be obtained.

Widely distributed oncogenic factors other than viruses also threaten species in nature, and selective pressures for resistance are likely to be operative with regard to susceptibility both to carcinogenesis and to progressive tumor development. The evolutionary considerations discussed for viral oncogens probably apply as well in many respects to other cancer-causing stimuli.

Etiological participation in at least some human cancers of chemical and radiological excitants similar to those blatantly carcinogenic in laboratory animals appears to be beyond dispute. It may be anticipated, accordingly, that the antigenic behavior of many human neoplasms is not entirely dissimilar to that of experimental neoplasms intentionally induced by chemical and physical means. The qualifications and reservations that limit the validity of laboratory tumors of viral causality as models of neoplasia in nature hold true for all experimentally incited neoplasms. Nonetheless, the marked success of immunological intervention against some chemically and physically, as well as against virally, induced experimental neoplasms affords grounds for hope that intelligent manipulation of host immune mechanisms can aid patients with many forms of malignant disease.

2.3 "Spontaneous" Tumors, with No Obvious Viral Etiology[1] (Animal and Human)

Designation of a tumor as "spontaneous" is a declaration of uncertainty as to its etiology, and conveys no substantive information beyond the nonintrusion of the observer in its immediate causation. In referring to spontaneous neoplasia, the qualification must also be made clearly that tumors arising unprovoked in inbred laboratory animals may fall far short, despite their "spontaneity" and even where the hosts do not carry viruses of known oncogenic activity, of representing veracious analogs of growths appearing in outbred organisms, and especially of neoplasms that develop under the normal ecologic circumstances of the species.

As indicated above, many neoplasms occurring in the absence of any intentional manipulation by the investigator are undoubtedly triggered into being, at one or another step in the progressive deviation from normal, by chemical, viral, and other factors similar to those used experimentally as carcinogens. The conditions of experimental and spontaneous carcinogenesis effected by the same agents may indeed differ pronouncedly. It is likely, for one, that carcinogenic stimuli are experienced in nature in much lower amounts than are employed experimentally, and there is persuasive indication that protective immunogenicity of TAAs is proportional to the inducing dose of carcinogen [19]. Nonetheless, the proven immunogenicity of many laboratory neoplasms suggests that at

---

[1] Tumors arising with high frequency in experimental animals bearing viruses of demonstrated oncogenic potency are here excluded from the category of spontaneous neoplasms

least some spontaneous cancers may be studied within the same immunological frame of reference, even though their antigenic potency may be far lower. Other spontaneously occurring tumors may be the final outcome of somatic mutations or selective gene activation, and of epigenetic malfunctions which disturb normal growth regulation or lead to the formation of tissue environments particularly favorable to aberrant growth, without the impelling force of specific external agents; the defects in cell structure and deportment, probably cumulative, may occur accidentally, at random, or as foreseeable stochastic concomitants of certain physiological functions, aging, and degeneration. Mutational changes, regardless of what has triggered them, are often accompanied by altered cell antigenicities, as may be nongenetic deviations in the composition and assembly of cell constituents. It would be incorrect, in light of these considerations, to view spontaneously arising neoplasms as lying intrinsically beyond the pale of immunological reactivity.

Although some spontaneous tumors of animals seem incapable of evoking sensitization expressed by acquired immunity to re-challenge, and give no other ready evidence of immunogenic properties [164, 165], other do provide indication of tumor-associated immunogenicity [15A]. In some instances, this immunogenicity is evinced by the manifestation of specifically heightened resistance in the autochthonous or in syngeneic hosts, accompanied by the production of detectable effector cells or antibodies specifically cytotoxic to the tumor; in others, there is evident only an excitation of humoral or cellular responses apparently directed at TAAs, without attestation of a defensive value. For an increasing number of human neoplasms as well, production by the patient of antibodies and lymphoreticular cells with specific reactivity against the autochthonous growth has been documented (see citations above). Although the *protective* immunogenicity of the corresponding antigens on such human tumors remains to be defined, there are seen, not infrequently, persuasive ancillary indications of the import of immunological reactions for host refractoriness.

The commonly observed patterns of fluctuating opposition and susceptibility to neoplastic advances in the patient; the correlations sometimes ostensible between propitious clinical status and a histological complexion of the tumor site suggestive of active immunocyte attack [41, 43, 183, 232, 293, 406]; the occasional spontaneous regression of advanced neoplastic lesions, often following severe infections with agents known to potentiate immunological responsiveness [270, 354]; and the therapeutic efficacy, albeit still largely anecdotal and limited, of immunological intervention, all betoken the existence of host immunological and immune potentiality against spontaneous neoplasia. The evidence is, admittedly, indirect and circumstantial, and no single set of observations hinting at immune reactivity resolves the question of causality. Cumulatively, however, the natural history of at least some neoplastic processes in man as well as in animals speaks for active host defenses of immunological kind. The impression is borne out experimentally. The early observations of Brunschwig et al. [57] on neoplastic auto- and homotransplants in advanced cancer patients are a case in point. Although questioned on grounds of propriety of such human experimentation, the findings of these workers, supported and extended subsequently by other, unobjectionable techniques [42, 43], remain as premise for the operation of immunological resistance factors to a variety of human neoplasms, even in individuals with extensive tumor involvement.

It may be concluded tentatively that the data now available, although still scattered, intimate that spontaneous tumors are, on the whole, less likely to be strongly immunogenic than many artificially induced ones, but do not negate the ability of the host to mount some immunological and immune reactions against them. That these reactions often fall short – the progressively growing tumors presented to us clinically – does not vitiate the possibilities of bringing immunological resistance to a higher level by felicitous intervention.

Theoretical deliberation, too, favors the probability that most tumors, regardless of causation, express at least a measure of surface antigenicity associated with the neoplastic state [421, 423, 424]. Neoplastic cells generally differ to some extent from analogous normal ones in morphology and function, and many of the changes that come with neoplastic transformation involve the cell surface. Differences in architecture and behavior must be assumed to be rooted in alterations of the composition and arrangement of cell components; and even small changes in molecular structure, configuration, and topography readily confer new antigenic qualities. As long as our expectations remain reserved and focus on antigenic "handles" accompanying neoplastic transformations, rather than on prevalent, frank immunogenicities [161], we have before us an open field of investigation directed at immunotherapeutic goals – provided that the transformed cells possessing an earmark of altered antigenicity are also intrinsically susceptible to immunological attack.

It is evident, however, that the obstacles on the way toward these goals are very large. Efforts to benefit the cancer patient by immunological means start from a negative point of departure: the fact that he is a patient declares that the balance of interaction with the neoplasm which confronts him has already tilted against him. The factors responsible for the defeat of the host may be single or many. Genetic determinants, age, life experience, environmental circumstances at the moment, and the specific carcinogenic stimulus may act, separately or jointly, to create syndromes of immunological and other resistance insufficiency, systemically or at the site of tumor incipience; the dyscrasia may be aggravated by the developing tumor burden and by the consequences of conventional therapy. In some instances, rapidity of tumor growth may lead to an overwhelming, quantitatively, of host defenses that might have halted a slower-growing neoplasm. Host selective pressures on the population of neoplastic variants must always be suspected as bringing to the fore clones with evasive capabilities: in order to survive in a hostile tissue environment, tumor cells must "learn" rapidly to take advantage of lacunae in host resistance, to seek "staging sites" in localities partially sequestered from systemic immunological attack [419], to lose or modulate surface antigens which serve as targets for cytotoxic immune attack, to actively neutralize damaging antibodies and cellular elements of the host, and by any other means to escape potential immune surveillance. The occurrence of many such mechanisms of evasion has been described [212, 214, 442], and others may well be discovered; they are likely to include both adaptive adjustments to host hostility and the selection, probably sequential, of capable mutants.

On the other hand, no selective pressure is operative for host recognition and effective responsiveness vis-à-vis tumors that, at the present stage of phylogeny, develop late in life, beyond the period of peak reproductive activity; and selection for immunological, and any other, mechanisms of refractoriness is likely to be tenuous with regard to neoplasias that do occur earlier in life but only sporadically. Thus, for the majority of cancers that pose the clinical problem in man, exceptional idiosyncratic host immunological and immune failure indeed need not be invoked as a primary contribution to etiology. Rather, recognition and reaction faculties to TATAs characteristic of many neoplasms may have evolved only very imperfectly in the species, whereas, in contrast, each population of tumor cells is under strong selective pressure in each organism for avoidance and neutralization of those defenses that are brought to bear against them.

What are the modalities of immunological defense, spontaneously having some role in host–tumor confrontations in nature or brought into play by intervention directed at tumor cell structure and host reactivity? Different investigators currently tend to propose the candidacy of different key mediators and effectors of tumor immunity, cellular and humoral, but the claims seem dinstinguished as much by fashion as by convincing data coming from experimental analyses. It would appear that a variety of immunological defense mechanisms can be effective, to different extents and in different combinations and sequences for different neoplasms, and perhaps variously at different stages in a given neoplastic progression. In one or another circumstance, every known arm of the immunological response has been shown inhibitory or destructive for transformed cells, in vitro and in certain cases also in vivo. Included in this array of effector mechanisms are several classes of free antibody; K cells; natural killer (NK) cells; mature T lymphocytes, activated specifically or nonspecifically; macrophages as such, armed with specific antibody or T cell recognition factors, or activated nonspecifically by prior contact with antigens against which they had been specifically weaponed; and, at least in an auxiliary capacity, perhaps also the spectrum of other white blood cells [166]. Each of the immunocyte classes may be composed of multiple subpopulations with distinct (but changeable) predilections for effector, mediator, helper, and suppressor capacity. It is unwarranted today to advocate favorite candidates as the inclusive, central pillars of tumor immunity.

Even more formidable a task than precise characterization of the modes of antitumor reactivity in a given host–tumor relationship, at a given time, is the attempt to intervene selectively toward a strengthening of resistance. Immunological responsiveness must be viewed as an intricate network of positive and rescinding signals, and even in the clearest models of epitope–antibody interaction, we have only begun to learn the patterns of the labyrinthine maze. This holds true for both specific and nonspecific immunological stimulation: the chains of events that lead to magnified or depressed activity of any one arm of immunological responsiveness remain largely uncertain – and multiple processes are incited by any one form of manipulation.

In light of these considerations, what then are the most probable pathways to be taken in embarking on the still very tentative endeavor at immunotherapy of neoplastic diseases of man?

3 Approaches to Immunotherapy

Several distinct avenues of immunological intervention in neoplastic diseases, all still tenuous, present themselves within the strictures of very modest assumptions and very formidable difficulties. The present discussion centers on therapeutic intervention; however, some of the principles and eventualities to be weighed may be relevant as well, if appropriately applied, to immunoprophylactic attempts.

3.1 Active "Nonspecific Immunotherapy" with Immunomodulating Agents

The range and nature of the effects on resistance against progressive neoplasia which can be elicited by microbial and other "nonspecific immunomodulators" have been explored by the author in recent discussions of the subject [427, 429]. The heterogenous family of agents designated generically as nonspecific immunomodulators (or, adjuvants) can exert, under appropriate conditions, profound influence on immunological responsiveness to defined antigens, and on states of resistance against pathogenic microorganisms and tumor cells. However, those immunomodulators that have a demonstrated capacity to raise antitumor resistance in different models are still, for the most part, crude microbial entities of complex and undefined composition. Immunomodulator intervention in malignant diseases today is thus an attempt at altering in predicted, auspicious directions exceedingly delicate equilibria between multicomponental living interactants – host immunocytes and other cells on the one hand, neoplastic variants on the other – with Stone Age tools.

The specificness of immunological relationships, as of all biological relationships, must be defined with regard to both the origin and the consequences of events and with regard to both their mechanism and breadth. The lack of comprehensive information often makes such definition difficult; the difficulty is compounded by the imprecision with which the words "specific" and "nonspecific" are commonly employed. They appear in the literature not only to distinguish between reactions that are based and those not based on molecular identity, similarity, and complementarity – the sense in which the writer here resorts to the terms unless indicated otherwise – but also to connote narrowness or generality of phenomena. Mechanism and extent are clearly distinct aspects of interactions, however, and unless the vocabulary used to describe "specificity" and "nonspecificity" is used with thought, misleading apperceptions of the scope and nature of occurrences are readily introduced [423]. In fact, all possibilities and permutations of particularity and nonparticularity in interactions involving immunocytes must be entertained. Stimuli related to a given entity in chemical or physical properties may lead to effects that are correspondingly restricted, as well as to effects that are manifested broadly. For instance, immunization against tubercle bacilli with mycobacterial derivatives can incite antibody and delayed hyersensitivity responses directed at the parent bacterium, and also expressed against a variety of cells, taxonomically related or far removed, that bea common molecular determinants; at the same time, exposure to the "immunizing" stimulus can set into motion as well multiple changes in immunological and resistance capacity that are not limited to that molecular conformity. Conversely, the effects of treatment with a substance physiochemically unrelated to a pathogenic or antigenic unit can be very contained, displayed only toward that factor and a limited number of others – the therapeutic activities of some immunomodulators for a circumscribed number of microbial, viral, or neoplastic diseases to whose causative agents they are wholly dissimilar in molecular composition are a case in point – or they can be extensive. Neither the data at hand nor the space here available suffice for careful dissection of the molecular specificity and range of the immunotherapeutic findings and approaches elaborated in the ensuing pages; the caveat seems in order, therefore, that the reader is not relieved of responsibility to consider critically the implications of specificity and nonspecificity of all interactions considered.[2]

It is clearly apparent that the effects elicited by immunomodulators are many and diverse. Nonspecific and specific facets of both afferent and efferent arcs of immunologi-

---

[2]   A more detailed discussion of specificity and nonspecificity in biological interactions is presented in another, recent review article (Weiss, David W. Nonspecific Immunity and Cancer, In: The Mycobacteria: A Sourcebook, Wayne, L. and Kubica, G.P., eds., Marcel Dekker, Inc., N.Y., 1980, in press)

cal reactivity interact, overlap, give rise to each other sequentially or counter each other, and trigger as well manifold nonimmunological events. However, precise elucidation of immunomodulator mode of action in specified systems remains to be achieved; knowledge of the primary loci and molecular foundations of their influence on immunological and immune function is still far too fragmentary to permit a cohesive overview. The task of classifying immunomodulator behavior at present is thus doomed to imprecision from the outset, and any exposition of the options of "nonspecific immunotherapy" can only be essayed as categorization of the major areas and mechanisms of likely immunomodulator performance in the elevation of antitumor resistance. Nonetheless, effort at a rational grouping of the phenomena is obligatory if the potential opportunities afforded by the approach of nonspecific immunotherapy are to be realized. Even a modicum of understanding and control of the complex events which are accentuated, changed, or generated by immunomodulators is contingent on apperception of at least the outlines of their multifaceted activities. The ordering of phenomena is a condition as well as reward of their comprehension; arrangement and insight are reciprocal processes furthering each other, and must be undertaken even when each step can only be partial and hesitant. The following delineation of immunomodulator effects on resistance against tumors is proposed in this light.

3.1.1 Loci of Immunomodulator Influence on Antitumor Immune Responses

Emphasis is placed in this discussion of immunomodulator action on agents of microbial origin, which so far have shown, on the whole, the greatest efficacy in experimental animal test systems and have attracted the widest clinical attention; the MER fraction of tubercle bacilli [17, 27, 420, 422, 432], which has been a subject of the writer's interest for many years, is singled out to illustrate many of the points made. It is noted, however, that adjuvants of other origin may well impinge on host resistance to progressive neoplasia by similar mechanisms.

3.1.1.1 Nonspecific Potentiation of Specific Responsiveness to Tumor associated Antigens

This class of effects exerted by immunomodulators on host resistance has been considered the one most commonly manifested and perhaps the most important. It is also the one that appears most closely related to classical adjuvant behavior: ability to respond to specific antigenic stimulation by synthesis of antibodies or formation of sensitized effector cells is heightened, or skewed in one direction or another, by the modulating agent. The nature of the effects thus lies with a nonspecific magnification or redirection of specific immunological responses. In many instances, these would have been possible, at least potentially, even without recourse to the excipient agent, but to a lesser extent or in other avenues.

Several distinct possibilities of action can be entertained, taking place simultaneously or consecutively in a given immunological response [429].

The immunomodulator may alter the structure and topography, and thereby the degree and kind of immunogenicity, of cell membrane antigens. A variety of eventualities can be envisaged: adsorption of the modulator to surface constituents, or chemical interaction with them, leading to true or pseudo-haptenization; insertion of the agent into complex macromolecular or polymolecular determinants; deletion and substitution of reactive groups in the cell architecture; and other interactions bringing about innovation in the makeup, configuration, and charge of relevant antigens. The transmuted antigenic entity may thus become a more potent immunogen quantitatively, or one able to guide immunological responses in other pathways: new carrier-hapten and other recognition and helper circumstances may be created; tolerance may be broken toward the corresponding native configurations; and new equilibria of activating and suppressing reactions may be established. The common denominator of all these events is modification of sensitizing antigen itself. Once triggered into being, the new or shifted immunological reactions evoked may be perpetuated by, and expressed against, the unmodified TATA determinants as well.

Immunomodulators may impinge, directly or via influence on other cell types, on the maturation, differentiation, and replication of immunocytes and their precursors and affect the functionality of the mature end cells [415, 431, 436]. Profound impacts by mycobacterial and other microbial adjuvants have been observed on antibody formation, the generation of cytotoxic lymphocytes, and a spectrum of macrophage functions, even when the agents are introduced in vitro to immunologically reactive tissue or to isolated immunocyte populations and even where modification of antigen seems to be improbable [28, 33, 114, 115, 208]. For some adjuvants, effects on lymphoreticular cells themselves appear to be a major modality of immunoregulation.

In some cases, such central mechanisms of action can probably be explained largely or solely by a stimulated proliferation and maturation of reactive cells. Lymphocyte and macrophage expansion may be general, providing the organism with an enlarged immunocyte equipment including clones specifically programmed for the antigens in question. A more focused enlargement of the numbers of specifically responding cells may also be entailed, as suggested by experiments in which modulators have been seen to potentiate the generation of specific antibody producing and cytotoxic effector cells in vitro at dosages far below the threshold of any polyclonal mitogenicity [28, 32, 33, 115, 205]; it also appears that the mitogenic and adjuvant properties of at least some complex modulators reside in distinct molecular constituents [312]. Discriminative clonal expansion could conceivably include both lymphocytes with the appropriate antigen receptors, and macrophages carrying antibody or Ia gene products serving as the specific reactants. Selective deletion or functional impairment of suppressor cells, generally reactive or specific for a given antigen, may contribute to the increment in responsiveness [205].

Alternatively, the mode of action may involve qualitative changes in lymphoid and macrophage immunological functions: lymphoid cells altered in their receptivity to antigenic stimulation and in their faculties as helper, suppressor, and effector cells for specific humoral and cellular responses; macrophages in their auxiliary roles in antibody formation and in the generation of lymphocyte-mediated cellular immunity, and in their own capacity as specifically armed attacking cells. Alterations brought about by any one modulator in immunocyte morphology and physiology may involve more than one family of cells. The molecular grounds of such qualitative alterations and their relation to changed immunological function await clarification. Different mechanisms have been advanced [27, 175, 189], and it seems probable that they are induced and expressed at unrelated molecular loci in affected cells. For instance, the MER mycobacterial fraction elevates both the activity of macrophage lysosomal enzymes and the responsiveness of lymphocytes to diverse mitogenic and antigenic stimuli [121, 445]. Within the interlocking network of forward and reverse responses which makes up immunological function, departures from norms initiated at one location are likely, moreover, to lead to chainreactions of divergence.

Immunomodulators can also affect the circumstances of specific sensitization, in a variety of ways. The one best known in general immunology is the prolonged maintenance of antigen in tissues, the depot effect. Clearly one of the modalities of action of many modulating agents, depot effects might also be entailed in potentiated reactivity to tumor cells. Even when introduced at tissue locations removed from neoplastic foci, and before or after these develop or are implanted, modulators may eventually come into intimate contact with tumor cells or their antigenic moieties, and mediate storage effects. These may occasion delays in the degradation and clearance of TAAs from tissues, and facilitate a gradual ongoing release of antigens and thereby a sustained responsiveness.

Depot formation may involve more than a delayed disruption and breakdown of antigen. Complex interactions between antigen, adjuvant, and host tissues may be precipitated, and these may pertain to deviant cells with new antigenicities as well as to soluble antigens. One possibility is the facilitated sequestration, or "trapping", of antigenic entities by networks of lymphoid and macrophagic cells in lymph nodes or spleen [440], and perhaps also throughout the tissues where immunocytes accumulate and confront neoplastic invasion. Other circumstances augmenting such mechanical effects may develop in the course of reservoir establishement, as additional, independent mechanisms. For instance, many adjuvants are irritants, and the inflammatory and other responses which they provoke can produce new microenvironments in which the processing of antigen is altered and to which immunocytes may be drawn, perhaps with a preference of cell types that can mount immunological reactions of particular import for host resistance to a given tumor [4, 152]. Where the modulator is itself immunogenic, immunological responses against it may participate in forming novel tissue microenvironments. And the chemotactic properties of some adjuvants [352, 441] may aid the concentration of cells with defensive potency in the vicinity of neoplastic niduses.

3.1.1.2 Nonspecific "Spillover" of Potentiated Specific Responsiveness to TAAs

Nonspecific magnification by immunomodulators of specific immunological reactivity to TAAs may be manifested not only specifically, toward antigenic entities which incited sensitization, but also generally.

Antigen-reactive lymphoid cells, both B and T[3], can liberate an array of soluble substances – lymphokines – upon interaction with the provoking antigen. Macrophages, too, liberate upon certain forms of stimulation soluble factors with activities similar to those of some lymphokines [120]. Macrophages passively armed for specific reactivity against TAAs might be especially apt to secrete such substances; and the production of such agents may also be effected by the non-T lymphocytes responsible for antibody-dependent cell-mediated cytotoxicity, and by NK cells.

Lymphokines amplify specific immunological responses and extend them broadly and nonspecifically; indeed, the classical mediators of cellular immunity and related factors appear to play a larger role at times as the executors of immunological phenomena

---

[3]   Such liberation of lymphokines is well demonstrated for T_D, Lyl-positive, Ia-negative thymus-derived cells, and may occur as well for other subsets of T lymphocytes

than do immunologically competent cells as such. The soluble agents have various bearing on host resistance: they attract, hold in place, and activate immunocytes to nonspecific aggressiveness, and may also recruit them to specific reactivity; some are directly and non-selectively toxic for transformed cells; and some cause changes in tissue microenvironments of immediate or secondary consequence for the afferent and efferent arms of immunological responsiveness, and for tumor cell survival. The nonspecific activities of some lymphokines (nonspecific exept for apparent discriminations by the agents, and by the cells they activate, between normal and neoplastic tissues) thus represent a dimension of reactivity superimposed on specific immunological interactions.

Furthermore, specifically armed macrophages can undergo excitation to nonspecifc antitumor cytotoxicity at contact with the antigens to which their armament is directed [93, 101]. A variety of lymphoid cells, mature T, and cells with "spontaneous," "promiscuous," and "natural" cytotoxic propensities, may also acquire heightened nonspecific cytotoxic capacity for neoplastic variants following initial interaction with targets bearing other TAAs, in addition to direct, nonspecific actuation by lymphokine and related factors [37, 62, 159, 160, 162, 190, 338].

Nonspecific modulation of antibody production to TAAs may also be of significance to resistance not only by virtue of the increased or redirected production of molecules cytotoxic or cytostatic in their own right, or as the armament of otherwise quiescent immunocytes and of the chain reactions set into motion by the specific reactants: the mediators of humoral hypersensitivity, released or produced in consequence of antigen–antibody interactions, may also affect tumor resistance indirectly, as may the impact on tissues of antigen–antibody complexes. Little attention has been given the eventuality that such mediators and complexes could act positively in antitumor defenses, consideration having been focused on their immunopathological and blocking activities. It is not inconceivable, however, that changes in tissue conditions caused by these elements in the vicinity of tumor foci, and even systemically, can be unfavorable to progressive tumor development.

Alterations in tissue conditions which follow in the wake of anti-TAA reactions and their potentiation can affect tumor growth variously and nonimmunologically. The processes of inflammation set into play by originally immunological events, and of its containment and healing, can have large implications for the fate neoplastic clones. Inflammatory surroundings are in some circumstances hostile to at least some types of neoplasms, physiologically or by the agency of immunocytes stimulated nonspecifically to nonspecific tumor attachment and cytotoxic capacity [1, 111, 291, 414]. Infiltration of fibroblasts and other cells and ensuing capsule formation may sometimes serve to restrict mechanically the spread of potentially invasive tumor cells, or lead to avascular atrophy by interference with the regional blood supply and with tumor angiogenesis [105A, 141]. Conversely, it must be noted that some neoplastic cells may find inflammatory microenvironments supportive, and may find in stromal tissue composition nutrients, physical surfaces, and other elements requisite for growth and malignant deportment [323] as well as mechanical shielding from defensive immunological processes [350].

In magnifying and faceting specific immunological responsiveness against neoplastic cells, immunomodulators thus also expand appreciably the compartment of secondary, nonspecific, "spillover" effects which accrue from the meeting of immunological reactants with the relevant antigens.

3.1.1.3 Nonspecific Potentiation of Specific Immunological Reactions Against Antigens Other than TAAs

The release or production of mediators of cellular and humoral immunity and hypersensitivity, creation of tumor-hostile tissue environs, and conversion of innocent and of specifically reactive immunocytes to nonspecific tumor cytotoxicity could all be heightened not only by amplification of anti-TAA responses, but also by magnified and broadened immunological reactivity to various other antigens. It is difficult to evaluate in vitro the importance to antitumor defenses of modulator-potentiated responsiveness to antigens other than TAAs or, for that matter, of the nonspecific extensions of heightened reactivity to TAAs themselves. However, both classes of transaction could well carry a larger role in resistance than may appear at first sight. Numerous immunological reactions take place constantly in tissues, against a plethora of antigens (among which there are undoubtedly represented microbial moieties cross-reactive with TAAs). Many immuno-modulating agents also elicit specific sensitization against their own antigenic determinants, as well as adjuvant effects on "background" reactions and on the responses to tumor cells which are the intended object of the intervention. It may be nonspecific consequences of incidental immunological events, now exaggerated, which bring about heightened refractoriness to a neoplasm, not only modulated specific responsiveness to TAAs and the consequent spillover.

Immunological reactions and their modulation are likely, moreover, to have importance to the tumor host beyond the facilitation of attack against the tumor cells which initiated disease. Potentiated immunological responses may play a key role in resistance to new neoplasms which appear not infrequently in some cancer patients, perhaps in consequence of the immunosuppressive or otherwise carcinogenic potentials of conventional treatment or of the intrinsically compromised immune status of the patient. Healing after surgery and exposure to ionizing irradiation is aided by certain activities of immunocytes. Immunological capability is clearly a decisive element in confrontation with pathogenic microorganisms, and protection "incidentally" bestowed by immunomodulators against life-threatening infectious episodes may be of major import to the total management of malignant disease.

3.1.1.4 Antigenic Cross-reactivity Between Microbial Immunomodulators and Tumor Cells

Widely scattered antigenic similarities of cell constituents, obeying no predictable taxonomic boundaries and overlapping animal, plant and Protista kingdoms, are a recognized phenomenon. Evidence has also accrued in recent years for a not inconsiderable cross-reactivity between a variety of microbial antigens and of determinants strongly expressed on tumor cells [55, 56, 259, 332]. The implications of these findings for an understanding of evolutionary development, and of the genesis of neoplastic aberrations, may be large, although an integrated view of their meaning hat not yet emerged. What is of direct interest to the present topic is the eventuality that some of the activities of microbial "adjuvants" do not, in fact, lie with a nonspecific modulation of specific responsiveness, but rather in effect with an immunization (or, hyperimmunization) against shared antigenic determinants; this consideration may also conceivably open the way for specific active or passive antitumor immunization (see below) by means of cross-reactive microbial entities [332].

Although it is doubtful that cross-reactivities between supposedly nonspecific modulator and target antigen can explain all or most of the influences of such microbial compounds on tumor resistance, the degree of their contribution is still to be ascertained. The possibility cannot be dismissed that microbial antigens are presented to the immunological apparatus in a uniquely immunogenic state (the "intrinsic adjuvanticity" of microbial moieties?), and that the specific sensitization thus effected by determinants held in common with TAAs is far more powerful than for the same etitopes located on the tumor cell surface.

3.1.1.5 Direct Nonspecific Activation of Immunocytes and Its Nonspecific Consequences

Agents with nonspecific immunomodulator properties may be capable not only of assisting the development of specific immunological responses to TAAs and other antigens, but also of conferring on lymphoid and macrophagic cells *directly* and nonspecifically heightend capacity to inhibit or destroy neoplastic variants. All immunocytes may be so affected, including NK cells [154] and perhaps also other lymphocytes with seemingly indiscriminate cytotoxic tendencies; it must be considered that immunomodulators may act not only as mitogenic triggers and otherwise as stimulators of physiological functions but, if in close proximity to the tumor cells, as the necessary "glue" for facilitating nonspecific cytotoxic attack [37].

Such effects must be considered apart from the potentiated participation of immunocytes in specific reactions which are triggered by antigen, and in their spillover, although the responsible mechanisms may be related. Thus, the mitogenicity of many modulators and their various effects on the membrane structure, enzymology, and other characteristics of immunologically competent cells may express themselves in new capabilities of the immunocytes both to take part in specific immunological events and to cause damage straightforwardly to neoplastic tissue with little limitation of specificity, by contact or by mediator release [37, 38].

An example is provided by the nonspecific excitation of macrophages to tumor cytotoxicity by macrophage activating factors (MAFs) liberated from lymphoid cells by various stimuli [101], among which direct exposure to immunomodulators is one. Recent work in our laboratories [114, 115] suggests that the excitation by MER of nonspecific macrophage cytotoxicity for tumor cells, and of better ability to deal with bacterial pathogens [113], is mediated by soluble B and T lymphocyte products released upon contact of the cells with the fraction. Other reported observations on immunomodulator activities lend themselves to similar interpretation: a mobilization of indifferent immunocytes to generalized antitumor contact reactivity, and to the production or liberation of substances which nonspecifically affect tumor cell growth and survival, without involvement of sensitizing antigen, antibody, or antigen-specific effector-cell receptors.

Lymphokines produced in tissue culture may find therapeutic application in the future [448], and their in vitro production may be facilitated by immunomodulators, acting directly on the cells of origin or acting as adjuvants to specific interactions between sensitized immunocytes and corresponding antigen.

Another intriguing possibility that has come under scrutiny is the possible production or release by immunocytes (upon one or another form of stimulation?) of factors that can abrogate the neoplastic characteristics of transformed cell variants and in this manner perhaps impede further progression of a neoplastic process [245, 317, 431].

3.1.1.6 Nonimmunological Loci of Action of Substances with Immunomodulator Properties

The common denominator of the multifaceted activities alluded to so far for agents pos-sessing immunomodulator ability is that the effects are exerted on immunocytes, or are mediated, amplified, and extended by them and their soluble products. The boundaries between "immunological" and "pharmacological" reactions are exceedingly uncertain, however, and it is apparent that the manifestations of many types of interaction between specifically sensitized effector cells and antibodies on the one hand and their cognate tar-gets on the other are truly pharmacological in nature, and may lack all immunological specificity. Nonetheless, phenomena brought into being through influences on immuno-cytes, or through actions exerted by immunocytes, may be termed, for convenience of classification, as immunological. Many of the categories of immunomodulator action undoubtedly fall within the scope of such a liberal definition. It must be considered, however, that the same substances that are capable of acting via the agency of immu-nologically reactive tissue may also elicit primary effects on cells and tissues unrelated to the lymphoreticular system [52, 380, 444]. For instance, microsomal enzyme function of pertinence to drug metabolism may be modified not only indirectly by modulators hitt-ing at lymphocytes and macrophages which then transmit effects to other cells, but also by the immediate action of the agents. Or, the irritant properties of many adjuvants can precipitate tissue injury and provoke inflammatory responses directly, and tumor cells may suffer injury as "innocent bystanders" of tissue changes that evolve with little primary dependence on the participation of stimulated immunocytes.

Nonimmunological lines of action may be initiated even by modulators of defined structure and recognized influence on specified cellular and molecular loci of immuno-logically reactive cells: the same, similar, or different alterations in cell morphology and physiology might be elicited both on immunocytes and on unrelated cell types. This is even more likely to be true for complex, undefined microbial moieties, whose distinct components may each cause separate effects, on different tissue systems. The fact that our attention is given to events played out on, or by, immunocytes must not obscure the possibilities of simultaneous changes in other cells and of their ultimate translation into revised states of host resistance.

3.1.1.7 General Comments

Several aspects and implications of this tentative arrangement of immunomodulator activities deserve accentuation.

Modulator-driven reactions that are distinct in locus, scope, and prominence for host resistance nevertheless share common mechanisms. The eventual classification of mo-dulator effects must therefore take into account not only modes of action, but also their place within the total scheme of host–tumor confrontations.

Some of the modalities and parameters of modulator influence on host resistance to progressive neoplasia are identical with those pertaining to classical adjuvant action on immunological responsiveness to defined antigens; others are different, and it is obliga-tory to consider the dimension of nonspecific immunomodulation independently for each distinct system.

Strong emphasis must be given to the likelihood that optimally efficacious employ-ment of immunomodulators will prove to require preparatory conditioning of the tumor bearer. Means may have to be sought for reducing or counteracting mechanisms by which neoplastic cells neutralize host defenses, for instance the rapid and continuous shedding of antigenic membrane constituents which can block specific immunocyte receptors [6, 34, 272, 296], elaboration of nonspecific blocking and immunosuppressive substances [184, 402], and production of enzymes which act on immunoglobulins and may convert intact, cytotoxic antibody molecules into fragments with enhancing activity [442]. Plasma exchange of the patient preceding active immunological intervention might be employed to lower serum levels of nonspecific obtruding factors of tumor and host origin, and of antigen, free antibodies, and antigen–antibody complexes that interfere with the attack on neoplastic variants by cytotoxically potent immune components [184, 195]. The concentration of some of these substances could perhaps also be lowered, at critical points in the therapeutic strategy, by subjecting the host to treatment with metabolic inhibitors. Constraint of immunological suppressor reactions might be achievable by injection of specific antisuppressor cell sera, already developed and shown effective in some murine tumor models (anti-I-J alloserum) [139], or of hormonal and chemical reagents that seem to abrogate suppressor cell activity preferentially [310, 320, 321]. It may also be given to overcome, transiently and in part, general or focused immunological deficiency of the host by preceding or conjoint administration of thymosine and thymosine derivatives [129], levamisole [374], and other immunorestorative and immunopotentiating agents. One or several of these measures together could be of signal aid when integrated appropriately into the schedule of immunotherapy, in elevating the baselines of potential host reactivity and of the degree of freedom from inhibitory influences.

The focus of this discussion has been on the positive influence of nonspecific immunomodulators on host defense against tumors. It is evident, at the same time, that nonspecific immunomodulation can also have adverse input on immunological capability and on states of resistance. Abundant evidence is available to show that optima (empirically determined) of dosage, route of administration, and timing of treatment with a given modulating agent often fall within narrow ranges, and that a variety of factors characterizing a given host–tumor relationship at the moment of intervention influence profoundly the nature of the results obtained.

Immunomodulators are capable of stimulating suppressor cell function and perhaps of inducing depression of host responsiveness by other means, in both nonspecific and specific directions [J.G. Bekesi 1978, personal communication; J.U. Gutterman 1978, personal communication; 17, 127, 142, 209, 302, 303, 311, 312, 319, 327, 358, 422]; they may steer reactivity to TAAs away from the formation of cytotoxic immune elements, precipitate circumstances of antigenic competition [142, 311], and contribute to local lymphoid center "overloading" and anergy [3, 105]; and they can be severely injurious to host tissues and thereby cause a variety of secondary effects inimical to resistance, unless employed in amounts adjusted individually to patient reactivity [285]. The negative purport of modulators might be accentuated by preceding defects in homeostatic regulation of lymphoid proliferation; it may reflect distortions of the same mechanisms that under optimal circumstances potentiate host defenses; and it may involve distinct modalities of counterproductive action. The impact of a modulator on the immunological apparatus can be multidirectional and mixed, even at the same moment, and should be viewed as a concatenation of immunological happenings of which some are beneficial, others indifferent, and still others deleterious to the capacity of the host to face challenge. Much futher insight into immunological behavior and into the potentialities of nonspecific immunomodulation is demanded before the interlocking phenomena of native and stimulated immunological responsiveness can be sorted out, and their meaning for host defenses defined.

Such insight has become a central necessity for the clinical application of information accruing in the field of tumor immunology. The pronounced therapeutic, and even greater prophylactic, efficacy of immunomodulators in many experimental tumor models holds out the promise that the agents can be employed with an appreciable measure of success in cancer patients as well. Therapeutic immunomodulation is a two-edged sword in the fullest sense of the term, however, and it is painfully obvious from the exceedingly sparse success attained so far in clinical trials with nonspecific immunomodulators that their use cannot be haphazard and indiscriminate, as has been the case very largely so far [426, 428].

Some of the likely reasons for the disparity in results obtained with immunotherapy in tumors of animals and in human neoplasia have been weighed recently by Hewitt and by the author in discussions of the relevance of animal models to clinical immunotherapy [164, 425, 428]. What appears probable is that major advances in the clinic may now be conditioned on the development of further basic information. The clinical urgency of human cancer is such that it may not be justified to bring immunological investigations in patients to a halt until more of the intricacies of immunological and immune responses are unraveled, and the opportunities for their potentiation discerned with a degree of certainty. What can be done today, however, is to base the design of clinical programs on principles of immunology that have begun to emerge, rather than on considerations pertinent to other treatment modalities; to record as precisely as possible the immunological and clinical changes effected; and to maintain awareness that our efforts will remain explorative and short of their maximum potentials for some time to come. By positing no unrealistic expectations, very modest results will encourage rather than dissuade further effort.

3.1.2 Nonliving Immunomodulators of Microbial Origin

Immunomodulators derived from microorganisms ubiquitous in nature, such as moieties of mycobacteria, gram-negative bacilli, and corynebacteria, appear a priori to hold intrinsic advantage over agents of other derivation. As indicated, all substances affecting immunological function nonspecifically can alter immunological responsiveness and host resistance both in favorable and unfavorable directions. When we turn to modulators obtained from common pathogenic organisms, however, it seems not unreasonable to assume a margin of safety. In the course of polonged phylogenetic acquaintance with such microorganisms, higher animals may have achieved a modicum of adaptation making for positive rather than negative responses to their presence as regards ability to resist frequent, phylogenetically ancient survival challenges. Progressive neoplasia, appearing prominently at the same stage in evolution as the "classic" vertebrate immunological mechanism, may well fall into the category of threats to species existence.

It might be anticipated, moreover, that prolonged phylogenetic exposure to microbial adjuvants has come to lead to their supportive participation in immunological reactions that carry roles in normal physiological processes, beyond defense against pathogenetic invaders [432], viz., in the clearance of effete body constituents, the release of pharmacological agents that maintain smooth muscle and vascular tone, and perhaps also in events entailed in reproduction and in the fixation of tissue and organ boundaries [40, 97,

233, 379]. There may be presumed to be in effect, therefore, a greater leeway in the range of positive responsiveness of animals to agents which are omnipresent in their experience and which have the power to affect basic physiological mechanisms. A case in point from our recent studies on the effects of various modulators on macrophage phagocytic and antibacterial capabilities is the finding that whereas many of the microbial agents tested exhibit strong and consistent excipient action, substances of other origin, such as thioglycolate preparations, are often suppressive.

Nonetheless, even microbial immunomodulators can incite deleterious influences on immunological capacity and on resistance to bacterial and neoplastic parasites, when employed in excessive amounts or at inappropriate times in relation to challenge (see above), and much care must accompany their clinical application, any margin of safety notwithstanding. It is apparent, therefore, that nonliving, standardized modulating agents should be developed for nonspecific immunological intervention in human disease, not only because they are far more convenient than living entities and cannot cause progressive infection, but also because they lend themselves to controlled, quantifiable administration, under conditions at least empirically ascertainable as satisfactory.

The accessability of standardized and stable, albeit still coarse, modulator preparations is a first step to the goals of isolation and identification of the active principles, their synthesis, and the molecular "thematic variation" aimed at creating safer and more efficacious analogs. The feasibility of such overtures is illustrated by experiments with purified mycobacterial cord factor [26] and by the recent studies of *Chedid* et al., *Ribi* et al., and others with breadkown products of acid-fast bacteria [11, 69, 70, 71, 72, 73, 74, 236, 304, 305, 422] and of *Westphal* and associates with endotoxin moieties [439]. Although many of the more purified of these materials lack convincing immunotherapeutic strength vis-à-vis neoplastic diseases, the way is open for attempts at increasing their potency, by polymerizing poorly active entities into larger, less rapidly degradable structures, attaching them to carrier molecules, and essaying alterations and substitutions of their known constituents. It appears not improbable that fully defined substances, their synthetic congeners, and combination products will prove to have much greater utility than the "first and second generation" microbial entities now studied, living and whole killed bacteria and crude heterogenous fractions.

3.1.3 Intralesional and Regional Versus Distal Immunotherapeutic Administration of Immunomodulators

Some investigators have taken a rather rigid position on the need of introducing modulating agents directly into neoplastic lesions or their immediate vicinity ("intralesional" and "regional" administration, respectively). Other workers have opposed this view, the author included [429].

There is no doubt but that intralesional or regional injection of some modulators is mandatory for immunotherapeutic efficacy against certain tumors. It is also apparent, however, that some adjuvants are effective when injected distal to a tumor, and even when introduction is into removed lymphatic drainage sites; systemic application of agents is perforce the rule in leukemic neoplasias – where immunotherapeutic intervention has had the most significant successes in patients until now [377].

On balance, there would seem to be little justification for a doctrinaire stance on this question, and, indeed, the same modulator may be effective when given far-removed from a tumor site against some growths and ineffective by other than intralesional or regional administration against others. For that matter, it may not even be possible to hazard generalizations for a given agent and a given type of neoplasm; the size and location of the tumor and a variety of individual host factors may be determinants of the most efficacious routes of injection. This circumstance is exemplified by data coming from work with the MER mycobacterial fraction.

In the transplanted hepatoma-guinea pig model developed by *Rapp* and his associates [298, 299], prophylactic injection of MER as early as 6 months prior to tumor challenge implantation, and at a site contralateral to the eventual tumor implant, affords complete protection to approximately half the subjects [411]. In syngeneic mice, distal and systemic prophylactic treatment is effective against a spectrum of solid and leukemic neoplasms [27, 420, 422], and the limited retardation of tumor growth exerted by the agent when employed therapeutically against several solid tumors is as great or greater when treatment is administered subcutaneously at a removed locality as when it is into the area of the growth [81]. In contrast, therapeutic intervention by MER against already established hepatomas in inbred guinea pigs seems efficacious only when treatment is intralesional or regional [412]. This condition was found to apply as well for Rous sarcomas developing in outbred chickens challenged with Rous sarcoma virus, both in prophylactic and in therapeutic test systems [248, 249].

It must be borne in mind that some adjuvants may indeed have to come into intimate contact with tumor cells, and perhaps simultaneously with immunologically reactive tissue – but that this probably takes place in many instances throughout the tissues and regardless of the initial portals of entry of agent and of tumor cells. It may thus be that repeated distal or systemic injections of a modulator, in large amounts, can give rise to the same circumstances as a single, limited injection given intralesionally. All possibilities of administration should be considered for modulator use in patients, and the stance of the investigator must be empiric at this time. Intravenous application of nonliving agents deserves careful exploration, assuring as it does wide distribution of the modulator and hits on tumor cell aggregates, as well as activation of dispersed lymphoid centers. It has been emphasized in the preceding sections that protective effects may be bestowed by the same adjuvant via distinct pathways of action. Effectuation of a broad distribution of agents in host tissues thus holds the advantage, theoretically at least, of covering multiple possibilities of therapeutic influence, and circumvents the often formidable difficulties or impossibility of reaching tumor foci by direct inoculation.

3.1.4 Combined Modalities of Treatment Including Intervention with Nonspecific Immunomodulators

The evidence available today, from both animal and patient studies, strongly implies that nonspecific immunotherapeutic intervention is most likely to be of benefit when it is coupled with conventional treatment [82, 176, 378, 450]. As will be pointed out below, this appears to hold true for passive as well as for active immunotherapy. On the other hand, there is also a prevalent risk of inimical influence, reciprocally, between treatment agencies.

The requirement for close integration of immunological treatment with other therapeutic modalities rests on a number of distinct considerations. For one, the principle of a preparatory or coincident debulking of tumor mass by surgery, chemotherapy, and radiation, allowing the immune mechanism to deal with less than an overwhelming number of neoplastic cells, seems generally valid, although it may not *always* be the overriding condition of efficacy. Occasionally, experimental tumor hosts and patients with far-advanced disease and large tumor burdens do respond to immunopotentiation [1A, 240, 262, 343, 422]. Much more often, however, the chances of immunological intervention in experimental models seem inversely proportional to the extent of neoplastic involvement, and although it may not be justified to withhold such treatment automatically where conventional reduction of tumor load cannot be effected, the strategy of such attempts remains germane: immunological responses are often inadequate or reach exhaustion when brought to bear against very large numbers of target cells, especially vis-à-vis well established, adequately vascularized solid tissues. TAAs in prodigious amounts may stimulate suppressor functions or otherwise steer responsiveness away from the generation of cytotoxic immune elements, perhaps especially so when the antigens, released from necrotizing tumor foci, are presented in soluble form; and excess antigen may saturate receptors on killer cells, alone or in complex formation with antibody [21, 307, 348, 393, 394]. Neoplastic tissue can also elaborate a variety of immunosuppressive and blocking factors, or direct host tissue toward the production of such intervening substances. The lessening of tumor load by recognized treatments thus facilitates variously the opportunities potential in the immunological sphere. In affording eradication of neoplastic cells differentially susceptible to each treatment, multiple intervention also serves to prevent or retard the establishment of clones strongly resistant to any one modality.

The interactions between immunological and other therapeutic manipulations are probably very complex and ramified, however, and are likely to evoke effects beyond mere summation of the tumor inhibition actuated by each arm, postponement in the selective prosesses leading to treatment resistance, and clearing of immunological lines of attack by the other efforts.

It has been suggested that intact, or potentiated, immunological functionality may be exigent for optimally efficacious chemotherapy [258, 297, 361], analogous perhaps to the requirement of host immune capacity for the satisfactory action of antibiotics in infectious diseases. A variety of mechanisms may account for this interconnection. For instance, immunological responses against haptenic drugs could influence directly their distribution and maintenance in the organism to the benefit of the tumor host, and mitigate their toxicities. Reactive immunocytes and their soluble products may also impinge on the activities of enzymes participating in drug metabolism, with a resulting accretion of more effective and more selectively tumor cytotoxic drug breakdown product. Recent findings showing that some systemically applied immunomodulators concentrate in the liver and there induce large histological changes support this possibility [150, 404, 447]. The possibility might also be entertained that immunological reactions which in themselves promote tumor growth can have opportune therapeutic end results within inclusive therapeutic regimens: neoplastic cells stimulated to proliferation can become more susceptible targets for concordant cytotoxic treatments.

Conversely, the release of TAAs from cells injured by drugs or by ionizing radiation could provide, *under appropriate circumstances* (that may vary widely for each host-tumor relationship), immunogenic stimuli particularly given to potentiation in therapeutic directions by parallel immunomodulation from without. Exposure to drugs and radiation can, furthermore, inhibit suppressor cell activities and other immunological functions of adverse consequence for resistance to progressive neoplasia [155, 258, 275, 355]; the likely significance of such selective effects on immunological reactivity becomes evident in light of the supposition that the immunological response toward a given tumor is commonly and simultaneously a composite of elements with cytotoxic, indifferent, and immunity-negating (tumor-protective and perhaps also directly stimulatory, and immunosuppressive) functionality, and that stress or de-emphasis on any one component can tilt the balance in favor of or against the host. Conventional therapy can also facilitate the emergence of more immunogenic neoplastic clones by causing temporary immune suppression, with a resultant heightening of efficacious responsiveness by the recovering host; and both chemotherapeutic drugs and radiation might elevate tumor cell immunogenicity by haptenization, direct modifications of TAAs, somatic mutagenesis of neoplastic populations, and activation of latent viruses.

Both conventional therapy and immunological activation can result in partial injury to tumor cells, and thereby make them more susceptible to lethal damage by the complementary treatment. Other modes of interrelationship can be envisaged for the recorded additive and synergistic input of conjoint therapy of malignant diseases that includes immunological measures, specific as well as nonspecific. There is the further reflection that combined management of a patient may permit a diminution of each component modality without sacrifice of global therapeutic accomplishment. The decrease in toxic side effects achieved by reduced intensity of intervention may be of considerable benefit to the patient as such, even if the levels of tumor cytotoxicity and cytostasis reached by multimodality intervention is no higher than that attainable with maximum single-agent therapy.

It is no less apparent, however, that negative effects can result from multifactorial therapy, and that constant, intelligent vigilance is required; such vigilance cannot be marshalled until there develops a much better understanding of the nature of host–tumor associations, and until there become available reliable tools of assessment of the fluctuating status of total host resistance capacity. Without careful interpolation of the parts of combined treatment modalities, the effects attained may be no better therapeutically than those accruing from moderate single-agent management, and they can be reciprocally antagonistic and frankly detrimental to the host. An array of mechanisms can be invoked as responsible for negative treatment interactions. The maintenance, distribution, and metabolism of drugs could be affected inopportunely by immunological reactions against the agents or against host tissues engaged in their processing. There is the cogent eventuality that other treatments may lead incidentally to a selection of tumor cell clones with greater refractoriness to immunological assault. Under inappropriate conditions, accelerated cell injury and death may give rise to a paralyzing or suppression-inducing flood of TAAs in the organism. Chemical agents and radiation can compromise selectively immunological functions of defensive as well as of inimical import to host resistance; and it has been shown that immunomodulators can at times exacerbate [353] rather than prevent [364, 454, 455] the immunosuppressive influence of chemotherapeutic drugs. Clearly, precise adjustment of all the paramenters of multiple treatment is essential if optimal end effects are to be achieved.

Chemoimmunotherapy and radioimmunotherapy must be viewed as therapeutic modalities subject to laws and constraints particular to each combination schedule, and distinct from those pertaining to single-modality treatment with the constituent agents. The nature, quantity, sequence, and timing of combined treatment must be weighed not only in terms of the actions that can be exerted separately by each modality on tumor cells and tumor host, but also in terms of the influence of each form of intervention on effects elicited by the other. It has been common experience of investigators that the efficacy of multimodality treatment is indeed governed by exacting provisions, often within very narrow optimum range. The limitations apply not only to the combination of different categories of therapy, but also to the employment of different forms of any one, including immunotherapy. The current study of Bekesi and Holland in patients with acute myelocytic leukemia subjected, in addition to standard chemotherapy, to hyperimmunization with neuraminidase-modified leukemic blast cells, administration of MER, or both kinds of immunological intervention is illustrative. There appears to be a greater prolongation of remission and life in patients receiving only the repeated specific sensitization than in those also given continuous treatment with appreciable quantities of MER; the joint immunological therapy seems markedly efficacious, however, when dosage and frequency of MER application are lowered [25].

The design of many of the even recently initiated human trials of immunotherapy in patients who are also managed by other modalities has been largely divorced from the considerations here alluded to. Only when data accumulate from investigations planned and executed in their light will it be possible to come to a blanced assessment of the contributions that might be made by immunological components of multimodality intervention in malignant diseases of man [247, 353].

3.1.5 Possible Advantages Inherent in the Nonspecific Approach to Tumor Immunotherapy

The data at hand are insufficient to permit decision on whether specific or nonspecific approaches to tumor immunotherapy hold greater promise. The clinical studies reported so far have been predominantly with nonspecific immunomodulators, mostly of microbial derivation. The therapeutic benefits gained have been very limited, few of the trials based on randomized concurrent controls yielding statistically significant results [377]. The failures could be ascribed as much to unsatisfactory design and conduct of the investigations as to intrinsic limitations of the agents employed, but the fact remains that experience provides no ground today for enthusiasm regarding the likely impact of nonspecific immunotherapy on human cancer. Moreover, some tentative clinical endeavors with specific therapeutic immunization have yielded impressions as suggestive of some efficacy as those obtained with nonspecific intervention [85, 172, 179, 240, 343]. A current study that deserves particular attention is the work of Bekesi, Holland et al. [24, 25, 171]: treatment of acute myelocytic leukemia (AML) patients with neuraminidase-modified AML blast cells appears to prolong first remission and survival at least as convincingly as any protection conferred in this or other malignant diseases by nonspecific adjuvant treatment.

Animal experimentation, too, has been largely focused on the nonspecific option, but some of the findings coming from various programs of specific tumor hyperimmunization have been no less striking than the performance of nonspecific treatments [19, 99, 179, 182, 342]. As discussed below, the assumptions that underlie immunization of tumor hosts with chemically, enzymatically, virally, or genetically modified neoplastic cells have a sober rooting in basic immunology, even in light of the probability that tumor-associated immunogenicity of spontaneously appearing neoplasms is minimal.

It is pertinent to question, therefore, whether accent should now be given to further explorations of nonspecific or specific modalities of immunological stimulation of tumor hosts. There do appear to be certain inherent advantages to nonspecific arms of intervention, and these argue in favor of a continued interest in this pathway despite the discouraging clinical record until now. Some of these advantages are cited in succeeding paragraphs, but with the clear reservation that the potentials of neither approach have been exhausted, that resort to both, jointly, may be requisite for maximum therapeutic benefits in some circumstances, and that imaginative research along both avenues remains warranted.

1) Nonspecific immunotherapy does not entail some of the formidable obstacles in the way of efforts at specific immunization, notably those encountered in the preparation of tumor cell vaccines.

Tumor tissue is often unavailable from the autochthonous patient, or available only in amounts too small to permit the making of sufficient vaccine. Autochthonous tumor cells may be requisite, however, where cross-reactivity between TAAs of histologically related neoplasms is weak or lacking. Moreover, the relevant antigens may be unstable. Procedures which assure complete inactivation of living tumor cells and of any oncogenic agents present are also likely to degrade antigens; introduction of vaccines not fully inactivated is a dubious undertaking, at best, for cancer patients, and is precluded for healthy individuals who might otherwise serve as donors of effector cells or of antibodies for passive/adoptive hyperimmunization. Recent observations by Bekesi, Holland et al. (to be published) exemplify the danger that allogeneic tumor cells may proliferate in the occasional patient who receives them as vaccine, even where the cells have been subjected to modifying treatment and even where the immunizing preparation proves safe in the great majority of recipients; sudden lapses in immunological competence by cancer and leukemia patients may be a major predisposing factor to progressive growth of allogeneic immunizing cells, but such deficiencies are difficult to diagnose in advance, and the eventuality of their occurrence cannot be ignored. Moreover, even where inactivation of allogeneic, and of autochthonous, vaccine preparations can be accomplished without degradation of TAA immunogenicity, the introduction of antigenic neoplastic tissue to the patient is accompanied by peculiar immunological risks, viz., receptor blocking of cytotoxic effector cells, formation of interfering antigen–antibody complexes, stimulation of specific (and perhaps also of nonspecifically active) suppressor cells, and induction of other deviations from defensive immunological capacity [393, 394, 460]. There is also the realistic possibility that immunization with tissues that express normal cellular antigens in addition to TAAs can precipitate serious autoimmune pathologies.

The pitfalls of induced departure from optimal immune function exist for active nonspecific as well as for active specific immunotherapy, but they may be even less predictable and less controllable for the latter, especially in view of the possibility that individualized vaccines may have to be used for each patient. The consideration that nonspecific immunomodulation with microbial moieties may have a margin of safety accruing from evolutionary adaptation has been indicated above. If it is indeed true that receptivity to microbial immunomodulators has evolved in a manner assuring some ongoing protection against microbial disease and incipient neoplasia, therapeutic employment of microbial derivatives may constitute salutary exploitation of a prevalent defense adjustment in nature. In contrast, organisms do not usually have to cope with large numbers of neoplastic cells until late in life and in the course of unchecked disease, and certainly not in the circumstances under which tumor tissues are presented to evoke hypersensitization. It is improbable, accordingly, that there have evolved safeguards for propitious immunological handling of massive amounts of antigens associated with the neoplastic state. And what evolutionary habituation there may have accrued for dealing immunologically with microscopic, nascent tumor foci does not necessarily furnish as well assurances for "appropriate" immunological responses to specific tumor immunotherapy.

2) The range of effects elicited by nonspecific lifting of the baseline of immunological responsiveness is wide, and such breadth of activity may be indispensable for optimally effective intervention in malignant disease. It is not improbable that tumor variants in metastatic aggregates express TAAs differently than do cells in the original growth; such differences could be individual for each metastatic lesion [102]. Immunological control of disseminated disease cannot be essayed, therefore, by specific hypervaccination with preparations of TAAs indigenous to only some of many tumor niduses. Nonspecific immunostimulation, on the other hand, could provide a broad umbrella of heightened reactivity against a spectrum of tumor-associated antigenic configurations, and thereby a degree of protection against dispersed foci of the same neoplasm, against clones undergoing further antigenic modulation within a single focus, and against multiple primary tumors and secondary growths which appear with some frequency in cancer patients, perhaps as result of immunological and other disturbances consequent to the first malignancy or its treatment. This consideration may apply as well to antigenically reactive *preneoplastic* cells [148, 232, 350, 416, 419, 435], responsivenes to which might be able to abort a malignant process in its incipience. The same protective umbrella could also extend to the ever-present, life-threatening hazard of infection in patients debilitated by neoplastic disease and conventional therapy. Indeed, many of the nonspecific agents now under investigation for cancer immunotherapeutic potency have been shown capable of bestowing marked protection on experimented animals agains microbial pathogens, and such activities are now also being recorded in cancer patients [27, 84, 422, 432, 433].

There is the hope, moreover, that integrated stimulation of a tumor-bearing organism with nonspecific immunomodulators and with specific TATAs, presented spontaneously in the course of the disease or administered as specific vaccine, may leave the host with greater specific resistance to recurrent growth of residual tumor foci than does stimulation by only specific means [339]. Nonspecific immunotherapy could thus provide a critical increment in the state of immunity devolving on tumor hosts in their confrontation with the neoplastic challenge – but only in certain circumstances. The interactions between specific immunity developing in the face of tumor challenge and the results of nonspecific immunostimulation are complex, and at indicated above, the results of combined manipulation can be indifferent or antagonistic as well as beneficial [25, 186].

3) Clinical attention has so far been given almost exclusively to *therapeutic* aspects of nonspecific immunomodulation. It is apparent, however, that the potentialties of this approach exist also for the prevention of future neoplastic disease in still healthy individuals, and indeed the magnitude of nonspecific immunoprophylactic effects achieved in experimental animals is generally greater than effects obtainable by nonspecific immunotherapy of already established neoplasms.

If some of the nonspecific immunomodulators now employed in cancer treatment are found moderately effective and safe, their eventual application to prophylaxis in normal individuals at high risk of subsequent neoplastic disease becomes justifiable. Intimations of successful immunological intervention during carcinogenesis or in the early, subclinical stages of neoplastic development have been adduced from animal models [227, 271, 416]. A variety of circumstances – family history, age, habitual smoking, industrial exposure, and other variables – contribute to the designation of high risk. If the human organism responds to nonspecific immunomodulators in a manner analogous to that of a variety of experimental animals, intervention prior to the emergence of frank neoplasia might prove signally effective in delaying its eventual onset and in reducing its incidence.

It seems far more difficult, in contrast, to engineer the development of specific prophylactic intervention. Any such attempt is predicated on the expression of prevalently cross-reactive antigenic determinants among each of the more common types of tumor. Although new evidence is indeed developing in support of earlier claims for the occurrence of such related determinants [53, 67], the frequency and generality of antigen-sharing by similar tumors is still unknown, and the facility of translating shared antigenicity to protective immunogenicity largely untested. There are also formidable technical and safety problems to specific prophylactic immunization with tumor cell vaccines directed against the development of unknown cancers, at indeterminate times, in a small proportion of subjects. Although, as discussed below, the advisability and feasibility of specific prophylaxis may not be ruled out entirely in some individuals in danger of developing particular neoplasms, this approach appears more remote than the induction of comprehensive protection by nonspecific stimulation.

4) The host of a progressively developing neoplasm is evidently an organism that has failed to mount satisfactory defenses against the challenging cells. Although this fact does not necessarily vitiate attempts to increase responsiveness by specific hyperimmunization or to close escape routes of the tumor cells from specific immunological attack, the efforts seem compromised from the start. Similarly, the normal individual standing at elevated risk of later neoplastic disease might also be one with smoldering immunological dyscrasia. It may be more opportune, therefore, to seek ways of a basic rehabilitation or reorientation of immunological strength, by nonspecific modulation, than to try correction of deficiencies by still more presentation of antigen, even if it be in an altered and more potently immunogenic form.

In summary, the emphasis here given to some of the advantages of nonspecific approaches to tumor immunotherapy is not intended to contraindicate further investigations of active specific stimulation of antitumor immunological reactions. Rather, the accent is offered in defense of intensified efforts at a therapeutic modality whose results have not lived up to the initial, although preponderantly naive expectations, and whose future is now threatened by at least partially premature disappointment. The avenue of specific therapeutic hyperimmunization has attracted less attention in recent years, certainly in the clinic, and, as elaborated in the succeeding section, it may lead to significant progress for all its accompanying dilemmas. Nonspecific and specific immunotherapy should be viewed at this point as alternative, and perhaps as complementary, options. No assessment of their relative import can be made until the outcome of expanded study is evaluated.

3.2 Active Specific Immunization with Tumor Cell Antigens

The preceding discussions have already alluded to principles of immunological function and host–tumor interaction that are pertinent to all modalities of immunological intervention in neoplasia. Accordingly, attention will here be focused on certain aspects peculiar to the modality of acitve specific immunization.

As already emphasized, the basic impediment to active therapeutic immunostimulation of patients resides in the attested inadequacy of the organism to meet the neoplastic challenge; added to this handicap at the start are the risks, also referred to above, which go hand-in-hand with introduction of vaccines derived from pathogenetic entities. Nonetheless, efforts at therapeutic vaccination of cancer patients have been ventured from the beginnings of experimental and clinical oncology, and are continuing to the present (see above); and it appears warranted to maintain these probes despite the difficulties entailed. A number of arguments can be advanced for the expectation of some success to focused attempts at stimulating immunological reactivity against antigens characteristic of pathogenic cells, neoplastic as well as microbial, even when these have already gained large footholds in the tissues of their host.

3.2.1 General Considerations

Neoplastic involvement of the organism may be for some time largely insular, and confined to immunologically sheltered sites; tumors may also actively create about themselves barriers of communication with the surrounding host tissues [177, 350, 419]. Stimulation by the primary tumor and by metastatic aggregates of systemic immunological responsiveness under such conditions may be minimal, as may be their accessibility to host defensive elements. Moreover, regional lymphoid centers may be inactivated or made specifically unresponsive to TAAs early in the confrontation. Introduction of the appropriate immunizing stimulus from without could circumvent such anatomical and physiological impediments, and when essayed by optimal route, amount, and schedule could be imagined to succeed where natural stimulation in the course of the disease faults. There are at least some analogies in the realm of host-microbial parasite relationships where extrinsic immunization, or hyperimmunization, is necessary to enable an infected organism to abort incipient pathogenesis or to recover from already frank disease.

It is perspicuously evident that all efforts at immunological intervention in neoplastic disease demand imaginative craftsmanship, to force a way past obstacles that have defeated more commonplace attempts. Thus, for example, it may be appropriate to try direct infusion of immunizing material into vessels leading to refractory tumor niduses and local lymphatic centers as a means of focal vaccination, mobilizing immune reactivity in situ where systemic stimulation is ineffective [191, 192]. And, as already indicated for nonspecific immunomodulation, careful attention must be given to the intercalation of all immunological treatment within overall therapeutic management, so as to prevent antagonistic and to favor additive and possibly synergistic action.

These propositions may have application to therapeutic immunization with unmodified neoplastic cells, and with unmodified bacterial-borne cross-reactive antigens. (There is the intriguing possibility of employing microbial preparations as antitumor vaccines, on the basis of shared antigenicities and in the hope that the common antigens might be more immunogenic as expressed by the microbial cell, more refractory to degradation, more effectively distributed in host tissues, or otherwise better capable of eliciting immune responses than when they are presented as tumor cell vaccines.) The considerations take on greater reality when applied to the modification and presentation of antigens designed to amplify immunogenicity and to favor those immunological responses of greatest value to resistance [30, 31, 109, 267, 280]. Not a few possibilities for effecting such modification present themselves, and for some there is already an intimation of practicality and efficacy in the clinic [24].

The recent experiments of Fish [104] deserve mention in this connection. It was found that a low-molecular-weight fraction obtained from 3M KCL extracts of a methyl-cholanthrene-induced mouse fibrosarcoma could offer solid protection against otherwise fatal simulated metastasis of the same neoplasm to a majority of syngeneic hosts also treated with subeffective doses of cyclophosphamide, even though the living tumor did not elicit appreciably heightened resistance to rechallenge following surgical removal of primary implants. In contrast, another methylcholanthrene-induced fibrosarcoma which did induce heightened resistance in animals following first implantation and removal did not yield a similar extract with immunotherapeutic potency. It thus appears that neoplasms that fail to exhibit protective immunogenicity when growing in compatible hosts may nonetheless possess protective immunogenic determinants, whose activities are displayed by partially purified tumor cell preparations in certain therapeutic circumstances. These observations might be of particular significance in light of the "poor immunogenicity" displayed by many spontaneous cancers as assessed in the more conventional tests, i.e., by ability of intact living cells to provoke heightend resistance against secondary implantation.

The approach to specific immunization should be not only with reference to activation of cellular immunological elements, but with a view to improved antibody formation as well. The concept that antibodies directed at TAAs are generally inimical, or at best indifferent, to the development of immunological resistance to tumors would appear to be dated. Antibodies have been shown to play a variety of direct and auxiliary functions in transplantation resistance, and their participation as well in cytotoxic responses to TATAs seems increasingly probable [10, 36, 149, 261, 265, 289A, 301, 313, 395]. Some molecular species of antibody may be capable of direct destructive action on tumor cells, and there is the growing body of evidence for the ability of antibodies to "arm," and thereby to invest with specific cytotoxic capacity, otherwise indifferent immunocytes of both lymphocytic and monocytic type [66, 93, 288]. It may not be wholly unlikely, moreover, that at least some of the "natural" serum factors found markedly toxic for neoplastic cells [395, 396, 397] are in fact specific immunoglobulins, or reactive substituent fragments, elicited in response, perhaps, to cross-reactive antigens of microbial or other derivation. Suggestive indications of a therapeutic function in patients of antibody molecules, even when passively administered and of xenogeneic origin, have been reported [85]. Some antibodies with "unblocking" activity can neutralize serum-borne interference effects [20].

Highly purified, specific antibodies, especially if of monoclonal hybridoma origin, may also find employment as vectors of cytotoxic agents: homing in on foci of neoplastic cells, the immunological ligands could selectively concentrate toxic chemial or radioactive isotopes in the immediate vicinity of malignant targets, and thereby elevate the desired cytotoxic effects while sparing normal tissues from excessive damage [8, 122, 123, 174, 313].

Beyond the possibilities of their lethal or inhibitory action on tumor cells, in themselves or as specific weaponry on lymphocytes and macrophages, antibodies may also contribute to antitumor defenses circuitously. Thus, Vaage has recently postulated the occurrence in some tumor models of the following sequence of host responses to neoplastic foci in animals not previously sensitized (*J. Vaage* 1978, personal communication; 398): Specific B lymphocytes are mobilized to the tumor from adjacent lymph nodes. Antibodies are produced that react with moieties of disintegrating tumor cells, and that may injure and kill some but not most of the living cells. Connective tissue reactions developing in consequence of the antibody-triggered damage and inflammation then attract T lymphocytes from adjacent blood vessels, a yet undefined category of "sentry" cells perhaps playing a prominent role in the T cell localization. Many of the T cells do not, in fact, interact directly with the tumor, but rather initiate at its periphery the formation of capsular cell layers, reminiscent of classical tubercle formation, which delimit and ultimately destroy the neoplastic mass. (There may also come into play in the scheme of defense gainst various neoplasms the phenomenon of natural, species- restricted attachment (NA) of nonspecifically activated T lymphocytes to a spectrum of other cells [111]. Activation of T cells to NA ability can be brought about both by initial antigen-specific interactions and by factors in the inflammatory environment of a lesion [112]. NA of T lymphocytes to tumor cells can contribute to the binding affinity between immunocyte and target [111], and thereby facilitate effectuation of injury by those T cells that do react specifically and directly with the neoplasm. Activated T cell NA to either tumor or stromal cells can have further amplifying action: in the presence of such attachment, the cytotoxic proclivities of third-party cells – monocytes and non-T blood lymphocytes – are potentiated [112]. The defensive impact of immunocytes accumulating "at a distance" from a tumor nidus [41] may involve the mediation of released factors that are directly inimical to the neoplastic cells, or that participate in the generation of unfavorable tissue microenvironments and the formation of mechanical barriers.)

Antibodies directed at tumor-associated antigens other than TATAs, and perhaps also at tissue products of nontumor origin in the vicinity of the neoplasm, could conceivably evoke a concatenation of diverse events unfavorable to tumor growth. Characterization of tumor and other antigens which can elicit any such protective host responses seems today a rather far-fetched undertaking, but one which nonetheless deserves thought – at a time when other clinical efforts in the field have been so frustratingly undecisive. An instance of apparently successful immunotherapy with antibody against nontumor determinants is provided by the experiments of Schlager and Dray [323] who found that guinea pigs could be cured of progressively growing syngeneic hepatoma implants by "injection into the tumor area, 6 and 16 days after tumor challenge, of antibody specific to fibrin fragment E (FFE), an essential component in the formation of a fibrin matrix considered to be important in tumor development".

Resort may have to be made to auxiliary measures for the facilitation of active specific immunization, similar to those indicated above for nonspecific immunotherapy.

Although viewed here in terms of *therapeutic* intervention, active specific immunization might come to have some role in tumor *prophylaxis*. Individuals exposed to certain carcinogenic stimuli in their environment, otherwise at high risk of developing particular neoplasms, or indicating upon diagnostic radioimmunoassay – a promising but still unproven approach to the early detection of cancer [136] – the presence of still subclinical tumor growth, could perhaps benefit significantly from specific immunization procedures, provided always that the same or related target antigens distinguish families of similar neoplasms [156] or occur as "universal" determinants on many tumors.

3.2.2 Modification of Tumor Cell Antigens

Various means which present themselves for modification of neoplastic cells with the aim of altering their antigenicities have been discussed recently [267, 280, 289], and need be cited here only in brief. The hope underlying all efforts at immunization with modified tumor cells, and with purified preparations of modified TAAs, is that the response elicited against altered determinants will be manifested against unmodified entities as well, or that the host organism will acquire the ability in the course of immunization to initiate reactions now targeted at the native structures. The focus of attention in this area has been on changes in the immunogenicity of TATAs, but similiar considerations apply to any other antigen to which immunological responses may be of value for host resistance, as indicated in preceding passages.

Diverse chemical reagents, including those with immunomodulator activities, have been employed to bring about either intrinsic changes in the composition or arrangement of existing cellular antigens, or their haptenization [86, 106, 277, 326, 359]. Such processing of tumor cells has provided specific vaccine preparations which have proven effective in inhibiting tumor development in various models [197, 200]. Treatment of neoplastic cells with certain enzymes and with mitogens can also raise appreciably their immunizing efficacy [340]; the ongoing clinical trial of Bekesi et al. [24, 25] with neuraminidase-treated AML blast cells may be cited as preliminary indication of the not inconsiderable therapeutic capacity of enzymatically modified cancer cells in man. Modification by chemical and enzymatic means can give rise to protective immunizing efficacy of tumor preparations even where the unmodified tissue has no, or only minimal, activity.

The mechanisms by which various modifications increase tumor cell immunogenicity may be identical with some of those mentioned above in explanation of immunomodulator effects exerted directly on neoplastic cells. Existing TAAs may be changed chemically and in physiochemical characteristics; they may be haptenized and then present novel antigenic structures. Previously masked TAA determinants may come to expression in consequence of modification-induced rearrangement of cell surface molecules. Immunogenically empowered and newly exposed TAAs may incite greater, more persistent, and qualitatively redirected immunological responses; weak TAAs may be invested with the properties of full-fledged transplantation antigens, capable of provoking immune rejection. The basis for energized immunity-evoking behavior of modified tumor cells is undoubtedly diverse, involving cross-reactivity of strong, altered with weak, native determinants; carrier-hapten and helper effects; abrogation of specific immunological unresponsiveness; shifts in differential stimulation of reactive and suppressive responses; and differences in stability, degradability, and translocation of antigens in host tissues. It appears probable that more than one distinct mechanism is operative concurrently in the arousing or strengthening of immunological responses of import to resistance against antigens that have undergone modification.

Several examples may be given of the profound influence of antigen modification with small-molecular-weight chemicals on the nature of immunological responsiveness. In experiments with sheep red blood cells (SRBCs) as the cellular antigenic entity and with the hapten trinitrophenyl (TNP) as modifier, it was found by Naor et al. that under different conditions of exposure, different amounts of the reagent remain bound to the cell membrane [239]. It was then seen that SRBCs that retain large amounts of TNP convert what would have been a strong primary antibody response against SRBC antigens to immunological memory mediated by T lymphocytes, without appreciable primary anti-body production. Moreover, the kinetics of memory to the modified SRBCs, as assessed by tests for antibody-dependent cell-mediated cytotoxicity upon secondary stimulation and by other assays, differ substantially from the kinetics of memory induced by untreat-ed red cells, with the reactions still directed at the same original cell antigens [193, 239, 268]. In contrast, various simple modifying substances can, in other circumstances of immunization, potentiate markedly the primary production of antibodies specific for the parent antigens [193, 239, 268]; and, under appropriate conditions, chemical modification of SRBCs can lead preferentially to cell-mediated immunity (delayed hypersensitivity) and away from antibody synthesis [239].

Studies conducted by us and by many other workers have demonstrated immunolo-gical consequences of similar magnitude, both cellular and humoral, for modification of neoplastic as well as of other cells with a variety of agents. There are clearly large implica-tions for host refractoriness against tumors to any appreciable deviation in type, extent, duration, and sequence of immunological responses to TAAs.

Modification of cell membrane antigens that are not tumor associated, and that do not in the native state participate in reactions of import to a tumor, can also bring about tumor immune responses. Alteration, haptenization, and exposure of such normal deter-minants may effect a de novo exposition of antigens cross-reactive with, and immunoge-nically more potent than, some of the transformed cell's TAAs. Beyond this, presenta-tion to the organism of strong tissue antigens, potentiated to immunogenic vigor by the modifying treatment, can be conducive to the actuation of immunological reactions against simultaneously experienced weak antigens, including TAAs. Although their mode of action remains uncertain, a variety of synergistic (and antagonistic) effects of combined immunization with distinct antigens have long been known. A prevalent, although not exclusive, mechanism with regard to tissue antigens could involve the dependence of some cell-mediated immunological reactions on products of the major histocompatibility complex [334, 456]; copresentation of two or more determinants could expedite responsiveness by overcoming recognition defects. Among other pos-sible explanations for a positive combination effect is the liberation of immunostimulat-ing lymphokines or of other "endogenous immunostimulators" in the course of immu-nological interaction with the stronger of a mixture of antigens. In causing the appearance of new, strong cell surface antigens, modifying treatment could facilitate such lymphokine effects as well as create a new and more effective gestalt for TAAs. Alternatively, the desirable presentational effect could be brought about merely by a reassembling of cell membrane constituents encompassing TAA entities, contriving res-tructured molecular configurations even without creation of new specific epitopes.

Treatment of tumor cells by physical means may offer an alternative to chemical and enzymatic modification, and could bring to pass a similar array of diversified mechanisms leading to bettered immunological responses [342]. At this time, only empirical testing can reveal what kind of modification will be most felicitous for a given tumor; resort to the same treatment, under identical conditions, has been found highly successful in amplifying the immunogenicity of some neoplastic cells and wholly ineffec-tive for other, even closely related neoplasms [197].

There have also been advanced possibilities of immunization with tumor cell prepa-rations and separated fractions not *intentionally* subjected to modification. Work with immunogenic tumor cell fractions holds the attraction that certain moieties may come to be implicated preferentially in the induction of immune responsiveness, and others in suppressor activation, thus affording opportunities for an a priori direction to sensitization. Among the preparations tested have been variously "inactivated" intact neoplastic cells and subcellular materials obtained by viral, osmotic, detergent, and other agencies of cell disruption [342]. The likelihood cannot be excluded, however, that relevant antigens are, in fact, modified by treatments yielding subcellular entities – an eventuality apropos as well for any vaccine formulated with adjuvant substances [304]. With regard to viral oncolysates, to which some investigators have recently given particular attention [342, 346], the contingency exists here, too, that antigenic changes may be induced by the virus.

Recent work in our laboratories by Naor and colleagues [110] signifies another possibility for procuring tumor cells with modified, and heightend, immunogenicity. YAC lymphomas freshly taken from hosts are incapable of eliciting states of heightened resistance against the living tumor, or of inciting the generation of cytotoxic effector cells; instead, the fresh neoplastic cells tend to provoke suppressor reactions. However, when they are placed in tissue culture, YAC cells rapidly display antigenic properties evocative of protective immunity in syngeneic subjects and of cytotoxic responses that can be measured in vitro; these responses are then also manifested toward the seemingly inert cells grown in the host. Whether adaptive or selective in nature, the appearance of new immunogenic potency upon in vitro passage may furnish simple and rapid means of achieving wanted antigenic modifications for some types of neoplasms. Differential expression of antigens by tumor cells grown in vitro and in vivo has also been noted by other investigators [64, 318, 443].

Viral heterogenization of tumor cells has been another instrument for the intentional supplementation of tumor cell immunogenicity [224, 225, 372]. As indicated above, infection with viruses can cause chemical and steric changes in existing histocompatibility and tumor-associated antigens, and can add a variety of new determinants to the cells – virion, virus-coded, and virus-derepressed – that could function as haptens, as carriers of native determinants, or as new epitopes which in close association with the original markers might elicit more effective responses against the combined molecular entities. New products appearing in consequence of virus action might also serve to increase the adjuvanticity of the infected cells. The approach of viral hetrogenization, and of possible heterogenization by other infectious organisms [91a], seems to deserve further exploration today; agents may be found or variants produced, with a selective preference for neoplastic clones, and with unique ability to induce in them the translation of minimal antigenicity to effective tumor-related immunogenicity.

Heterogenization of tumor cells may also be essayed by genetic hybridization [216, 220, 276], in the hope that addition to the TAA spectrum in question of allo- or organ-specific antigens, or of unrelated TAAs, will create new antigenic configurations of value to antitumor immune stimulation. An intriguing possibility lies with the use of some hybridomas [255], made from lines of neoplastic and other cells of known antigenic constitution.

In summation, review of the many eventualities for modifying and potentiating the antigenic structure of neoplastic cells leaves the impression that this remains a worthwhile approach to tumor immunotherapy, despite the vexatious difficulties inherent in all active specific immunization. Attempts at tumor cell modification must evidently be essayed with care, all such treatments also holding the risk of destroying immunogenicity and of affecting inimically other properties of TAAs requisite for their stimulation of resistance responses.

3.2.3 Other Possible Means of Specific Immunization

An avenue of investigation that deserves renewed interest is suggested by the repeated observations that some TAAs are determinants which also appear on normal cells, but predominantly during early stages of life. It also appears that the same embryonic and neonatal markers are expressed by a variety of tumors. It is conceivable, then, that specific antitumor immunization, prophylactic as well as therapeutic, could be attempted with normal fetal tissues [19, 66, 253; see also citations above]

A number of such attempts have indeed been reported, but in view of the failure of some of the preparations tested to induce heightened resistance to tumor challenge or to hinder the progressive development of established growths, the approach has been largely dismissed as futile. The negativism is not founded, however. Failure at protective immunogenicity of some well-characterized preparations – such as the "carcinoembryonic" antigen(s) (CEA) – nor more vitiates the conceivable efficacy of other antigens of this biological type than does inadequacy of any other one or several substances condemn automatically an entire class. The finding that some fetal and neonatal antigens do, in fact, have the capability of inducing immune responses to tumors supports this reservation, and further exploration seems justified, with stress on the use of immunomodulators, antigenic modification, and possible attachment of the determinants to carrier entities. On the other hand, the risks of causing autoimmune disease (AID) by employment of fetal antigens may be especially pronounced. As intimated above, some such determinants may continue to be expressed by certain normal cells (in particular, undifferentiated precursor cells of various tissues), albeit in small amounts; hyperimmunization could arouse strong and damaging responses in adult organisms against ontogenically archetypic markers to which tolerance is not absolute, the more so if the vaccinating antigens are introduced in modified form. Stem cell function may be especially prone to such injury [289A]. It must be asked, therefore, whether the dangers of AID stimulation, which indeed attend all immunization with tissue vaccines, are forbidding, or whether they can be limited by judicious adjustment of the immunization program and by resort to known methods for managing AID pathology. Limited AID may be a tolerable price for the elicitation of antitumor responses, and the question may thus have to be posed individually for each immunizing preparation and for each host–tumor circumstance.

Vaccines composed of (inactivated) oncogenic viruses might also find eventual clinical application, prophylactically and therapeutically, although this approach is heavily impeded by the difficulties of ensuring abolishment of all oncogenic activity while safeguarding antigenic properties. Nonetheless, the prominent representation of virion components among many tumor sensitizing and target cell determinants encourages the effort. So does the consideration that continued presence of oncogenic viruses may sometimes be requisite for ongoing neoplastic disease progression, even after the initial transforming events have taken place [250, 300]. Relapse in human leukemia following what is taken to be total therapeutic eradication of all leukemic cells may also involve the agency of carcinogenic viruses, especially where the "recurrent" neoplasia appears in restorative hemopoietic implants of donor origin [381]. An early experimental indication of the immunizing capacity of inactivated viruses against "spontaneously" appearing, virus-induced neoplasms is provided by the author's experiments with formalin-treated, purified mammary tumor virus preparations in inbred mice [59]. It must be taken into account that the procedures of virus inactivation might also cause modifications of relevant antigens, and that it is the antigenic alteration which in fact facilitates protective immunogenicity.

Cell antigens appearing in consequence of infection with oncogenic viruses may appear on still-normal tissues after ingress of the agent [91]. It may be possible, according-ly, to utilize infected noncancerous tissue for vaccination, thereby assuring presentation of a complement of virus-associated determinants and avoiding the problems inherent in the use of already frankly neoplastic tissue. Experiments in mice have pointed to the practicality of this approach, at least in experimental models [91].

A still largely unexplored question is whether cells exposed to chemical or physical carcinogenic stimuli but not yet endowed with plain neoplastic characteristics, similarly express antigens identical, or cross-reactive, with some of the TAAs which appear on the fully transformed variants. Some affirmative indications for tissues still seemingly nor-mal or in the early stages of premalignancy have been provided [231, 350]. If such early emergence of relevant antigens does indeed occur not uncommonly in some nonviral carcinogen-tissue interactions, it may be given to produce polyvalent vaccines against some types of neoplasms from still-normal tissues following their *antigenic trans-formation*, provided that the range of purported tumor-individual antigenicities of many such neoplasms is not too broad or that there occur additional common antigens. Affir-mative answers should give special impetus to prophylactic intervention, in individuals known to have suffered extensive exposure to carcinogens with a predilection for the generation of certain neoplasms in given demographic and environmental circum-stances.

3.3 Passive and Adoptive Immunological Intervention

3.3.1 General Considerations

The salient preference for attempts at passive and adoptive immunological intervention in neoplastic disease resides in the facility of circumventing circumstances that hinder the organism's defensive capabilities. Failure to control progressive disease can clearly be of multiple origin. The immunological ingredients of shortcomings in resistance have been referred to throughout this volume; they are reasserted here in emphasis of the approach of nonactive immunotherapy.

Genetic and acquired factors can make for general inadequacy of immunological and immune function; and more specific incompetencies may exist in those clones of immunocytes and other cells which bear the burden of resistance against a particular challenge. Where host defensive cells are inherently capable of executing resistance functions, a variety of specific and nonspecific factors produced by tumor or host can interfere "peripherally" with resistance. Peripheral interference may not be manifested evenly throughout the tissues of a tumor host. The well-described phenomena of con-comitant immunity are evidence that success and failure at tumor inhibition may concur in different tissue localities vis-à-vis neoplastic foci of different size and in different microenvironments. The many experimental and clinical observations that removal or in situ destruction of one tumor focus can have important consequences for the fate of others, both stimulatory and inhibitory [118, 284, 341, 360, 370], similarly attest to the supposition that circumstances in addition to those that define central, intrinsic resistance potentials can impinge importantly on host–tumor interaction. The impression is reinforced by fingings the immunocytes obtained even from hosts with far advanced neoplastic processes can display, in isolation, strong cytotoxic activity against the autochthonous tumor, despite the evident failure of the intact organism to contain the neoplastic process [237, 252, 264, 344, 405, 406], or that such cells can take on cytotoxic ability in culture once they are freed from in vivo blocking mechanisms [251A].

Even where they commence without impediment, immunological events in vivo must always be considered as taking place against a background of homeostatic controls which limit them in time and extent, and whose evolution is a mandatory condition of metabolic economy and of the prevention of self-destruction.[4] Varients of normal progenitors, neoplastic cells can well be imagined to escape, like their normal counterparts, the cytotoxic activities of immunocytes programmed for their recognition. The equilibria which assure that normal cells normally escape immunological attack [119] while effete and deviant ones must of necessity be eliminated, might not be so finely attuned as to disallow all neoplastic variants the opportunity of escape by preemption of normal homeostasis [266]. Subject to constant selective pressure in their host, populations of neoplastic cells are likely, moreover, to develop active mechanisms for avoidance and neutralization of the instruments of host defense [212, 214]. To direct the intact organism's immunological responses through a labyrinth of safety controls and toward effective attack on tumor cells without causing major damage to very similar normal tissues, and to negate simultaneously all the mechanisms of "sneaking through" by the neoplasm, would be an arduous task even if our insight into the machinery of immunological function were far more sophisticated than it now is. The pressure to develop immunological weapons against cancer has given impetus, and perhaps justification, to the empiric immunotherapeutic efforts that have been undertaken, but we should cherish few illusions as to the probability of great accomplishment by active host immunization or immunomodulation in the dark.

There are thus strong grounds for a turn to the alternate pathway of passive and adoptive immunological intervention [99, 180, 313, 382]. Although, too, still highly empiric, this approach infers undeniable advantages, especially with regard to the employment of cytotoxic effector cells and antibodies that are produced in tissue culture. The advantages indeed pertain largely to the possibilities of in vitro generation of antitumor immune elements, and the topics of passive/adoptive therapy and in vitro sensitization will be treated, accordingly, as one.

3.3.2 In Vitro Generation of Cytotoxic Effector Cells Against Tumors

A number of investigators have demonstrated the feasibility of in vitro sensitization (or, "generation"; "education") of lymphoid cells to specific cytotoxic reactivity against neoplastic cells [96, 128, 131, 132, 194, 201, 207, 208, 237, 263, 286, 309, 322, 329, 331, 384, 387, 405, 452]. Because such work represents a major undertaking in our laboratories during the past several years, regard is here given to findings made by our group, in illustration of

---

[4] The interesting observation of Lewis et al. might be noted, that human cancer patients can indeed mount strong immunological responses directed at the idiotypes of antitumor antibodies (and effector cells?), one reaction thus negating another of potential defensive value [244]

the development of this field of investigation and of the resources inherent, at least in principle, in the strategy of passive/adoptive immunotherapy.

Under idealized tissue culture conditions, experimentally determined and carefully controlled, large numbers of potent effector cells[5] are generated by normal lymphoid tissue (spleen, lymph nodes, blood, and peritoneal washings) of mice and humans within less than a week in the presence of inactivated tumor cells (one-way mixed lymphoid cell–tumor cell cultures; MLTCs); such sensitization can be effected even against neoplastic cells which evoke little or no immune response in the intact host [201, 202]. Lymphoid cells from tumor-bearing hosts can also be sensitized in culture, or their already evident reactivity increased, but the conditions and manifestations of effector capacity may be decidedly different for normal and for presensitized responder cells [132, 237, 263, 330, 402, 405, 452].

The tissue culture microenvironment must be set precisely for each responder cell–tumor cell system [201, 207, 329]; minor changes in one parameter of the MLTC system – such as ratio of responder lymphoid cells to stimulator tumor cells, total number of cells in the culture, volume of the medium, and size of the vessels – often demand changes in other parameters, and standardized conditions found ideal for the education of lymphoid cells of given origin against a given tumor may be unsatisfactory for other lymphoid cells and other tumors. Despite the demanding nature of the in vitro sensitization conditions, however, the production of cytotoxic effector cells in a controlled system is highly consistent and predictable, once the parameters are fixed.

In a variety of mouse leukemia, lymphoma, and solid tumor models, sensitization can be effected in vitro (employing lymphoid cells derived from individual donors, or pooled cells) vis-à-vis both syngeneic and allogeneic neoplasms [208, 286, 309, 322]. Nonreactivity of pooled or single-donor mouse responder cells has been encountered rarely in our studies.

In man, peripheral blood white cells (PBWs) obtained from a high proportion of patients with solid tumors and from leukemia patients in remission can be sensitized effectively against autochthonous tumors [131, 132, 237, 344, 405, 452], even where no cytotoxic activity is displayed prior to MLTC incubation. The PBWs of some patients, however, remain anergic, failing to develop cytotoxicity even when allogeneic tumor cells of the same type are utilized as stimulators [330, 402, 405]. Responder cells from normal healthy allogeneic donors undergo in vitro sensitization even more frequently, against a variety of human leukemia and solid tumor cells, although occasionally a population of both responder and neoplastic stimulator cells proves ineffective. In vitro sensitization to autochthonous tumors can be potentiated, or brought into being where it otherwise fails, by addition of allogeneic stimulator cells to the autochthonous neoplastic stimulators [237, 452, 453], a finding reminiscent of the excitation of cellular immunological responses to weak tissue antigens concurrent with induction of reactivity against stronger cell immunogens.

Recent findings in our laboratories coming from "crisscross" experiments, employing one human neoplasm for in vitro sensitization and a spectrum of histologically related and unrelated neoplasms as test target cells, indicate that allogeneic recognition

---

[5]   In the discussion on in vitro sensitization, the term "effector cell" is employed to denote lymphoid and monocytic cells with cytotoxic reactivity manifested after in vitro culture; the term "responder cell," lymphoid cell populations prior to sensitization

and reactivity is manifested against specific and cross-reactive TATAs, not only against histocompatibility markers [207]. Such specificity appears against the presumed background of strong (and in the experiments conducted so far, uncontrolled) HL-A antigenicities. These results are in keeping with the experimental findings of other investigators which have documented the recognition of individual TAAs in the presence of other, potent, virus-determined antigens; they may also be analogous to the observations of Wainberg et al. [409, 410] on autochthonous preference of recognition (although interpretations other than prominence of individual-specific reactions within a heterogenous framework of reactivities have been advanced for this work [334]).

In syngeneic murine test models, cytotoxic reactivity of in vitro sensitized effector cells is often, although not invariably, highly specific for the neoplastic target cells which were employed as stimulators in culture [208, 286, 322, 384]. Where cross-reactivity has been evident, it might be largely attributable to antigens associated with common viral agents [335]. In allogeneic mouse systems, cytotoxic reactivity is displayed against the corresponding tumor cells as well as against normal, mitogen-transformed lymphoid cells of the same histocompatibility type [202]. However, recent studies with responder lymphoid cells from mice primed with allogeneic lymphoma and then sensitized further in vitro suggest that populations of cytotoxic effector cells may be mixtures of subpopulations, of which some are directed toward H-2 alloantigens and others against TATAs; these subpopulations of effectors can be purified and enriched [89]. The parallel generation of distinct effector clones with alloantigen and with tumor-associated specificities has also been noted by other workers [14].

Work in progress in our laboratories suggests, moreover, that certain chemical and physical treatments of allogeneic tumor stimulator cells may reduce or abrogate their ability to provoke cytotoxic anti-histocompatibility antigen responses in MLTCs, while leaving intact their provocation of such responses against TATAs [254]. A preliminary finding of similar interest is that solubilization of tumor cell membranes may be, under certain conditions, more damaging to the immunogenicity of normal transplantation than of tumor-associated antigens. If it becomes clear that (some) TAAs retain protective immunogenicity upon treatment which cancels or lessens the immunogenicity of normal tissue antigens, evocation of anti-self reactivity following either active or passive immunization might be reducible to acceptable levels. It may then prove possible to favor generation of the desired antitumor responses in vitro even in allogeneic MLTC combinations. Furthermore, Devens et al. have found that cultures of splenocytes from mice primed with allogeneic tumors tend toward the emergence of effector cells bearing specificity for TAAs and against that of effectors directed against alloantigens [89].

A major effort is now necessary to ascertain precisely the degree and limits of specificity of cellular cytotoxic reactivity brought about in vitro, taking into account the likely conjoint and variable expression of TAAs shared by neoplasms of the same etiology and of the same histological type, of antigens specific to the individual tumor, and of a spectrum of histocompatibility determinants.

It remains probable, nonetheless, that some effector cell clones directed against normal self-constituents will be represented in lymphoid populations following in vitro sensitization, despite all attempts to make sensitization conspicuous for TATAs. Anti-self reactivity may be manifested not only where sensitization is in allogeneic MLTC systems, but also where the cell combination is autochthonous: representation of lymphoid cells with anti-self reactivity has been demonstrated within the lymphocyte complement of normal individuals [80]. Incubation of lymphoid cells in the presence of even autochthonous stimulator cells may thus lead to enlargement of the anti-self clones and to their "activation." It seems possible, however, to reduce further the risk of graft-versus-host (GvH) reactions ensuing from therapeutic employment of sensitized effector populations by selective deletion of anti-self clones from the inoculum, as discussed below.

The mechanisms underlying in vitro generation of specific effector cells remain to be clarified. The very rapid appearance within lymphoid tissue cultures of a high proportion of specifically reactive cells seems difficult to explain within any framework of clonal selection of preexisting catalogues of cells genetically programmed for diverse reactivity. It may be that selective replication of specifically cast clones existent within the lymphoid pool of normal animals, and induced changes in conformation and functionality of the relevant cell surface receptors, are not the only operative modalities; the "sensitization" event might involve as well a transfer of specific information or immunological equipment to other cell populations in the responder mixture [79]. Although these basic questions await resolution, experimental evidence for the ability to achieve massive production of specifically cytotoxic effectors within several days of contact with stimulator cells has become indisputable.

Data now developing in our laboratories indicate that the effector cells obtained by in vitro sensitization, both in syngeneic and allogeneic murine and in autochthonous and allogeneic human cell combinations, are predominantly T lymphocytes, although some effector participation by macrophages has not been definitively excluded. It is also possible that NK cells, and populations of lymphoid cells representing intermediate stages of differentiation, play some part. Suggestions have been offered that NK cells may be, in fact, immature T cells [145, 159, 160, 437, 438], or K lymphocytes armed with certain "natural" antibodies [159]. Some NK as well as mature T cells may be considerably specific in their reactivities [145, 308, 437], the latter perhaps partly in consequence of antibody (or other factor, Ia or Ir?) arming; such arming could be envisaged to occur during in vitro education, by T cell agents or by antibodies produced simultaneously in responder cultures consisting of mixed lymphoid cell populations. Moreover, contact with corresponding antigen can effect an increased and perhaps more focused NK activity [62, 162, 190], although it is uncertain whether the increment represents clonal expansion, adaptive changes in a constant number of competent cells, or arming with antibody or other recognition factors; another possibility lies with the nonspecific stimulation of NK activity by interferon or other lymphokines [159, 363] released in the course of adjacent immunological interaction. In any event, it has been shown that strong NK reactivity becomes evident in cultures of human lymphoid cells after several days, especially when the media contain fetal bovine serum or certain other antigens [190].

Macrophages appear to cary out a necessary helper function in the generation of cytotoxic T lymphoid effectors, at least in some of the murine and human models examined (E. Kedar 1978, personal communication; 407). On the other hand, Kedar has recently observed that thinning out of phagocytes from the responder cell population, by means of colloidal iron and magnetic removal, appears to enlarge NK activity (E. Kedar 1978, personal communication), perhaps because of elimination from the MLTC of nonspecific suppressor activities. Further study is required to define precisely, in each sensitization system, the contribution of the various lymphoid and macrophagic cell populations to responder activity and to effector function, both specific and nonspecific (see below).

In both murine and human test systems, maximum first sensitization is achieved within 5 to 7 days of culture [201, 207]. At that time, most or all of the mitomycin C or radiation inactivated tumor stimulator cells have disappeared. There is a rapid decline in effector cell numbers or activity after 1 week. However, addition of a new pulse of inactivated stimulator cells to cultures maintained for several weeks after primary in vitro sensitization rapidly evokes renewed reactivity, suggestive of a typical secondary response as seen in vivo [202]. There is also intimation that the therapeutic efficacy of second-response murine effector cells may be greater than that of first-response effectors [75].

The cytotoxic capacities of murine effector cells generated in vitro have been measured by in vitro assays [201, 286, 384], notably ^{51}Cr liberation from labeled target cells, by Winn neutralization and protection tests [75, 202, 309, 316], and by assessment of the therapeutic proclivities of the effectors in animals already bearing neoplastic isografts [60, 75, 203, 204, 313, 386]. Only in vitro tests have been applied systematically so far to human effector cells, barring some tentative and still anecdotal attempts to employ them therapeutically in patients [180, 252, 313, 328]. There appears to be very close correlation in some systems between the in vitro and in vivo activities of murine effector cells sensitized in culture [203, 204], thus permitting prior in vitro determination of reactivity of cells to be employed therapeutically. Recent experiments have indicated, however, that distinct subpopulations within the same sensitized cell culture may be responsible, at least in certain test models, for cytotoxicity as measured in vitro and for therapeutic activity in the tumor host. Further work is in order toward the characterization of differentially reactive effector cell populations, and their enrichment for therapeutic purposes.

Under optimal conditions of in vitro sensitization, both syngeneic and allogeneic murine effector cells produced in culture can effect lysis of 90% or more of the corresponding tumor target cells in vitro (3-h ^{51}Cr release assay, at effector/target ratio of 10/1–30/1), and can give categorical protection in Winn assays against otherwise invariably fatal inocula of living tumor cells, even where challenge injection is intraperitoneal or intravenous (E. Kedar 1978, personal communication; 204, 205). When such effector cells are employed therapeutically in mice bearing leukemia or lymphoma isografts, without parallel chemotherapeutic intervention, they frequently slow the neoplastic process and prolong significantly the life of the animals. Cures are effected only in a small proportion of the subjects, however [60, 75, 203, 204]. In contrast, combined treatment with chemotherapeutic agents and effector cells commonly leads to permanent cure in 90% or more of the animals, even where the untreated controls succumb within a few weeks and chemotherapy alone is curative in less than half the mice [75, 96, 204]. Therapeutic results of this order are obtained with syngeneic and with allogeneic effectors, and with numbers of allogeneic cells below the threshold of GvH disease induction [204]. Even allogeneic effectors which display strong cytotoxicity in the in vitro ^{51}Cr release assay against *normal* (mitogen-transformed lymphoid) target cells of the same H-2 type as the leukemia stimulator cells in culture, as well as against the same neoplastic cells, are highly effective in passive chemoimmunotherapy without usually eliciting discernible symptoms of GvH or other pathology [204]. Where GvH syndromes are noted, they are often transient and moderate [51].

PBW effector cells from cancer and leukemia patients and from normal human donors also exhibit strong reactivity in the chromium liberation assay, but the magnitude of the effect is often somewhat lower than that attained with mouse effector cells, and the optimum conditions of MLTC incubation appear more narrow and demanding.

Mice surviving Winn or therapeutic assays in which either allogeneic or syngeneic effector cells sensitized in vitro were employed for neutralization of the tumor inoculum are solidly resistant to massive rechallenge with the same neoplasm several months later [202, 208]. An unexpected finding has been the altered sensitizability of splenocytes taken from such survivors several weeks to months after performance of the test. Such spleen cells show no cytotoxic activity when tested directly. Upon in vitro sensitization with inactivated neoplastic cells of the same type, however, effector cells are obtained with considerably greater efficiency in the chromium release, Winn, and tumor therapy assays than is seen for effector cells derived from normal donors and then incubated in MLTC [203, 204]. This heightened reactivity, and the acquired resistance of the host, do not seem attributable to any specific immunization of the animals in course of their experience with the tumor inoculum in the original Winn test: the degree of specific immunity that can be bestowed by active immunization with these leukemic cells falls far below that observed in the present circumstances [124, 125, 187], and control experiments with mice challenged with the living neoplasms, not given effector cells, and cured by chemotherapy revealed no such heightened refractoriness or splenocyte sensitizability. Moreover, recent experiments indicate that animals injected only with allogeneic or syngeneic in vitro sensitized effector cells, without any neoplastic cells, gain similarly potentiated splenocyte sensitizability as well as heightened resistance to tumor challenge. Specific immunization would thus appear to be ruled out, unless one were to invoke the existence of a "super" TAA (see, for instance, 9A), activated to unusual protective immunogenicity in the MLTC sensitization process. Neither can the changed reactivity of Winn assay survivors be attributed to a long residuum of effector or memory cells where these were allogeneic. Rather, it appears that the effector cells employed originally in the Winn procedure affect in some manner the test animals' own lymphoid tissue, transferring information and "recruiting" host cells that then respond in magnified manner to further tumor exposure, in vivo and in vitro. Data pointing to comparable enlistment phenomena have been reported by other workers [78, 79, 383]. Experiments are now under way in our laboratories toward definition of this apparent recruitment, with a view to the possibility of utilizing subcellular effector cell fractions for therapeutic purposes.

3.3.3 Potentiation of the In Vitro Generation of Cytotoxic Effector Cells

It has proven possible to increase the cytotoxic activity of in vitro educated effector cells, both human and murine, more than a hundredfold, by certain treatments of stimulator tumor cells and of responder lymphoid populations, and by resort to immunomodulators in the MLTC [197, 199, 205, 206]. It must be emphasized that attempts at amplification of in vitro sensitization are accompanied by considerable variability, and that the parameters of every excipient measure must be carefully defined and fixed for each responder cell–tumor cell system.

Treatment of mitomycin C inactivated neoplastic stimulator cells with chemical reagents (trinitrobenzenesulfonic acid, iodoacetamide, trinitrophenyl) or with enzymes (trypsin, neuraminidase, papain, bromelain) often magnifies the sensitization process appreciably. Frequently, however, the same reagent potentiates the response of similar lymphoid populations to one modified tumor but not to another [197]. Inactivated enzymes are ineffective. The modes of action of stimulator cells treatment in vitro may well be the same as those responsible for heightened immunogenicity of modified tumor cells in the intact organism; the possibility cannot be excluded, however, that some of the modifying agents also exert selective effects on helper, suppressor, and effector functions of the responder cells.

Enzymatic treatment of responder cells prior to MLTC incubation, and of sensitized effector cells, can also magnify the cytotoxic end result [206]. Among the mechanisms suggested for these effects have been the bringing into more prominent relief of receptor molecules of potentially reactive cells and the release of substances with nonspecific adjuvant activity, or of recognition factors capable of endowing other cells with specific helper or effector capacities.

Supplementation of the MLTC mixtures with microgram quantities of MER commonly results in a categorical augmentation of specific cytotoxic reactivity, whereas larger quantities of the agent are strongly suppressive [205, 207, 436]. In some cases, MER is, in fact, requisite for the elicitation of specific sensitization. For instance, peripheral blood lymphocytes from patients with lung carcinomas fail to undergo sensitization in the presence of the autochthonous or allogeneic tumor cells, but develop high reactivity, as seen by in vitro ^{51}Cr liberation tests, when small amounts of the immunomodulator are introduced to the cultures [199].

The addition of MER must be effected within the first 48 h of culture, suggesting that the agent acts on the early events of sensitization [205]. It should be recalled in this connection that some immunomodulators may be able to enlarge the complement and/or functionality of NK [154] as well as of mature T lympoid cells, directly or via the intermediary agency of interferon or other lymphokines released by other cells; such release may be, in turn, a direct influence of the adjuvant, or may occur in consequence of stimulated immunological reactions, perhaps against the adjuvant agent itself.

The presence of MER in splenocyte cultures containing fetal calf serum has been found to reduce or abrogate the generation of nonspecific suppressor activity [198, 205]; however, quantitative considerations suggest that such action is not the sole factor responsible for potentiation of specific in vitro sensitization.

In addition to heightening specific sensitization in the presence of stimulator cells, supplementation of the culture medium with MER also gives rise to a degree of seemingly nonspecific cytotoxic activity, apparently T cell in nature, manifested toward a broad spectrum of syngeneic, allogeneic, and xenogeneic target cells (but not against normal cells of the same histocompatibility type) [205, 206]. Such nonspecific reactivity is evoked by the agent even in lymphoid cultures devoid of any specific stimulator cells. Work is under way to determine whether distinct lymphoid cell populations are responsible for the potentiated specific and for the apparently nonspecific cytotoxic reactivities, and whether macrophages participate to any appreciable extent in the latter.

On the other hand, the suggested existence of cross-reactivity between some TAAs and some microbial moieties raises the question whether potentiation by MER is indeed wholly nonspecific, and indicates, moreover, the possibility of employing microbial antigens as specific stimulators for the in vitro production of antitumor cytotoxic effector cells or antibodies [332, 333].

An excipient effect on in vitro sensitization is also brought about by polyethylene glycol [206], a compound known to substitute for macrophages in the potentiation of lymphocyte activities in vitro [315]. Examination of other nonspecific immunomodulators and of substances with known helper proclivities in the development of cell-mediated immunity is now warranted. The findings already at hand leave little doubt as to the large potential of such agents for amplification of effector cell production; recent experiments by us have already confirmed the stimulating activity of muramyl dipeptide and of other mycobacterial fractions [206].

The in vivo cytotoxic activity of sensitized lymphoid cell populations can be concentrated by enrichment of specifically reactive clones on bovine serum albumin, and perhaps also on other, gradients [206]; the numbers of such enriched cells required to achieve the same therapeutic effects exerted by unprocessed populations are considerably reduced. Removal of nylon-adherent and histamine or Fc receptor-bearing cells at the beginning of incubation are additional means of enlarging and congregating cytotoxic capacity. Pretreatment of donor mice with cyclophosphamide or hydrocortisone also heigthens sensitizability of their lymphoid cells [206, 310, 321]. Suppressor cells have been given popularity as the central limiting factor to immunological resistance against malignancy, and the greater capacity of lymphoid cells to undergo cytotoxic education in culture following such donor pretreatment or selective responder cell depletion is currently ascribed to removal of specific or nonspecific suppressor clones or their precursors; it seems premature, however, to posit this as the only explanation.

Recourse to a combination of several distinct techniques for potentiating in vitro sensitization provides cumulative magnification of reactivity [206]. To what extent each form of manipulation serves to increase and concentrate the numbers of effector cells, to elevate the cytotoxic proclivity of each cell, and to free potentially reactive cell populations from suppressor influences requires further analysis.

An important finding has been that tumor stimulator cells and lymphoid responder cells, as well as effector cells after in vitro sensitization, can be cryopreserved for prolonged periods without discernible loss of reactivity [202, 207]. Such stability under carefully defined conditions of cryopreservation has been seen repeatedly for human as well as for mouse tumor and lymphoid cells; a major logistic problem in the planning of passive or adoptive immunotherapy of human patients with in vitro sensitized effector cells thus seems to have been solved, although the possibility cannot yet be excluded that preserved effectors may have some impairment of vitality and therapeutic capacity in man.

3.3.4 In Vitro Production of Antibodies and Its Potentiation

The possible role of antibodies in immunological resistance against cancer, directly or as the ordnance of neutral lymphoid cells or macrophages, has been discussed above. Primary synthesis of antibodies in vitro and the elicitation of anamnestic responses are well established, and there are large similarities in the conditions and kinetics of the generation of antibodies and of cytotoxic effector cells in tissue culture [33]. Possibilities exist, accordingly, for producing in culture large quantities of specific immunoglobulins with desired antitumor activity, either by creating circumstances preferentially favorable to the synthesis of given molecular species of the ligands or by their later separation from heterogenous antibody pools.

Recent work has shown that MER exerts not only a polyclonal mitogenic effect in vitro on B lymphocytes [28, 32] (and perhaps on T lymphocytes as well [260]), but also a specific proliferative stimulus for cells making antibody against antigens added to the primary cultures [29]; even when the amount of MER employed falls below the threshold of polyclonal mitogenicity, large increments occur consistently in the numbers of specific plaque-forming cells produced and in the titers of free antibody. Work now in progress suggests that the presence of MER, and perhaps of other immunostimulators, may give preference to the manufacture of one or another class of antibody in certain lymphoid cell populations, a finding in line with earlier observations in vivo on the highly selective influences of the agent on immunological responsiveness [30, 31].

Major advances toward the unrestricted availability of specific antibodies may come from the work of Steinitz et al. [357] on virus-induced immortalization of clones of antibody-producing cells. It may prove possible to effect the establishment of monoclonal cell lines producing immunoglobulins of specific class as well as of specific idiotype, thereby providing a variegated armory for passive use. Although not yet applied to the production of antibodies specific to TAAs, there appears to be no counterindication in principle to the inclusion of such antigens in the range of specificities of B cell immortalization; initial sensitization to antibody production in vitro, against purified TAA preparations, may facilitate the effort by amplifying the number of relevant clones for viral transformation. A second approach to the genesis of monoclonal antibody-producing cell lines lies with the creation of appropriate hybridomas.

3.3.5 Possibilities and Problems of Clinical Application

The strategy envisaged for passive/adoptive immunotherapy in the human patient is analogous to the plan of treatment in experimental animal hosts of neoplastic cells, and can be outlined in principle as follows:

Lymphoid cells will be obtained from the peripheral blood of patients during remission or disease-free interval, at a time when no neoplastic cells appear to be present in the circulation. Alternatively, allogeneic lymphoid cells from normal healthy donors or from patients apparently cured of similar neoplastic disease may be used as responders for in vitro sensitization. If further investigation pinpoints the types of responder and helper cells engaged in the tissue culture generation of antitumor cells, the relevant populations of cells will be employed in place of whole PBWs.

Tumor stimulator cells, fresh or cryopreserved, will be of autochthonous patient origin, or from another patient with similar disease. If further research provides justification, resort may also be made to established tumor cell lines (bearing in mind the eventualities of loss of relevant sensitizing antigens and other undesirable changes in long-cultured cells), and perhaps to purified TAA preparations. It may prove possible, in addition, to evoke antitumor cell sensitization by pooled allogeneic normal cells, on the supposition that (some) TAAs may be identical or cross-reactive with (some) normal histocompatibility antigens of unrelated individuals; indeed, the superiority of such sensitization of autologous lymphocytes from leukemia patients over that induced by the neoplastic cells themselves has been reported [453].

The stimulator cells will be inactivated, and they and the responder-effector cells treated by one or more of the several means described above for potentiating sensitization; MER or other immunostimulators may also be introduced to the cultures. After 5-7 days of primary, or 3-4 days of secondary, MLTC sensitization, the effector cells will be havested, purified by gradient separation so as to concentrate the effective cytotoxic population, and cryopreserved; additional work is necessary to ascertain whether effector cells obtained by secondary sensitization are indeed more satisfactory for clinical use.

At the "appropriate" time, the effector cells (autochthonous cells for "adoptive" and allogeneic cells for "passive" therapy) will be thawed and injected into the patient, systemically or in some instances perhaps directly into blood or lymphatic vessels leading to solid tumor foci [191, 192]. Initiation of passive/adoptive immunotherapy might be most appropriate at a point when the patient shows signs of incipient relapse or disease progression, or perhaps while he is still in full remission. The timing, quantification, and frequency of passive/adoptive treatment, and the nature and scheduling of conjoint active chemotherapy and, possibly, immunotherapy, will have to be defined empirically by clinical investigation.

Preliminary experimental and subsequent clinical trial is also in order to explore the possibilities of passive therapy with antibodies produced in vitro, as such or as the armament for (defined) populations of lymphocytes or macrophages.

As indicated in preceding paragraphs, treatment strategy of passive/adoptive intervention is straightforward and its theoretical advantages over active immunological intervention notable. Neither patient nor other responder cell donor need be subjected to any procedure of specific vaccination or nonspecific immunomodulation, with the attendant difficulties and risks. When introduced in sufficient quantities and at the opportune times, the immunological reagents produced in vitro, cellular and/or humoral, are anticipated to "home in" on the neoplastic target cells remaining in the patient, and to effect their destruction or growth inhibition.

Conditions can be set in culture for the rapid generation of cytotoxic effector cells and antibodies even against very weakly immunogenic neoplasms. As further knowledge accrues, it may be possible to define and utilize optimum combinations of purified and enriched helper, responder, armament-producing, and potential effector elements. The immunological microenvironment in the reaction vessel can be idealized by trial and error, and a large degree of freedom secured from the limiting complexities of immunological responsiveness and its homeostatic controls in the intact organism. Restrictions placed on defensive host reactivity in vivo by a spectrum of blocking and neutralizing factors of host and (metabolically active) tumor origin are obviated; and any central host immunological dyscrasia can be circumvented by employment of reactive allogeneic lymphoid cells.

Repeated emphasis is in order of the probability that all procedures of antigen modification and immunological potentiation can have obverse consequences when undertaken in vivo. Immunomodulators can thwart desired immunological reactions under circumstances which may not be predictable at the start; a case in point are the recent reports that T cells isolated from mice treated with complete Freund's adjuvant have deleterious effects on tumor immunity in vivo and fail to undergo sensitization to cytotoxicity when incubated in culture with antigenically reactive stimulator cells [127, 302]. Modified tissue antigens are apt to induce immunological responses strongly damaging to related native tissue, perhaps especially in subjects with defective immunoregulatory function. Restraint of such inimical effects seems far easier to achieve in the empirically constructed, and expendable, in vitro culture systems than in the unpredictable immunological matrix of the whole organism. And where objectionable populations of cells are produced in culture – effector cells with GvH proclivities; specific and nonspecific suppressor cells – it may be possible to remove them selectively [12, 48, 89, 246] or at least to coordinate the timing and extent of passive/adoptive therapy so as to reach an optimum balance between therapeutic and negative side effects.

Auxiliary measurs which may have to be taken to assure the functioning of passively administered immunological weapons have been described above.

In practice, however, the problems and obstacles to the application of passive/adoptive immunotherapy are formidable, and even though steps can be envisaged for their resolution, therapeutic success in man is still in doubt. The accomplishments attained in inbred mice bearing laboratory tumors provide a clear impetus for clinical exploration, but there is no assurance that the closely defined conditions for efficacy in murine test models can be duplicated in the human patient, and not even preliminary information is as yet available from the clinic to presume that passive/adoptive immunotherapy in man will prove to be more than another, albeit interesting, disappointment.

It may be very desirable to use autochthonous effector cells. Their immunological and physiological compatibility with the tissues of the patient to be treated favor their retention upon reintroduction for the longest possible time, and the dangers of GvH pathogenesis would seem to be minimized. The possible expression of autochthonous preference of reactivity may constitute another advantage. Where adequate numbers of autochthonous responder cells are not procurable directly from the patient, it might prove feasible to enlarge the relevant T cell populations considerably, by enrichment of sensitized PWB cultures with factor(s) released by lymphoid cells upon mitogenic stimulation [49, 126, 314]. Further expansion of desired clones might be attainable if means for true immortalization of effector or memory T cells could be developed; experiments on viral infection of T lymphocytes are in progress in a number of laboratories with this aim [94, 95]. This has proven a difficult task so far, T lymphocytes apparently lacking receptors for appropriate viruses, but experiments currently under way with Sendai virus as a linking agent and with RBC ghosts carrying EBV as inserting vehicle may overcome the difficulties (D. Johnson 1979, personal communication).

Serious short comings of autochthonous effector cells must be weighed, nonetheless, apart from the question of availability. They may be incapable of undergoing effective sensitization because of impaired immunological competence for one or another reason, and they may have an intrinsic inability to respond well to TAAs only marginally different from normal self-constituents. Neither can freedom from the problems of GvH and host-versus-graft-reactivity be taken for granted. Clones with anti-self reactivity can come to the fore in culture, where they are removed from blocking or tolerance-inducing influences, and may then encounter little hindrance in repopulating, and injuring, the autochthonous recipient. Conversely, lymphoid cells may undergo changes during in vitro maintenance and growth which could cause them to be recognized as foreign upon return to the original donor and to suffer accelerated elimination [60, 204]. There must also be entertained the danger of reimplanting, systemically and in large numbers, autochthonous neoplastic cells that may already be present among supposedly normal responder-effector populations, or that appear in consequence of new, "spontaneous" transformations in vitro.

The danger of such neoplastic variants finding a foothold in patients is considerably reduced for allogeneic responder-effector cells, even in individuals whose immunological capacities are below normal. It may not be entirely inconceivable, moreover, that arsenals of allogeneic antitumor T effector cells could be prepared and stored for wide use, by expansion of the reactive clones with mitogen-induced factors or by immortalization procedures, if the supposition is indeed in order that cross-reactivity exists between the TAAs of some human neoplasms related histologically or etiologically. Even if such clonal amplification should fail as practical measure, the logistics of allogeneic responder/effector cell availability seem far less intractable than is the case for autochthonous patient cells.

On the other hand, the projected application of allogeneic effector cells could be compromised severely by host-versus-graft and graft-versus-host difficulties, the latter especially in patients whose immunological deficiencies are marked; and by the risks of inserting foreign pathogenic microorganisms, oncogenic agents, or other pathogenetic factors. It would appear probable that very large numbers of effector cells must be given to patients, repeatedly, in order to effect significant tumor destruction or inhibition. For instance, the number of neoplastic cells remaining cryptic in AML patients in "full" clinical and hematological remission may be as high as 10^9, or higher; by analogy to mouse therapeutic models, rather staggering numbers of sensitized effector cells may then be required to elicit clear therapeutic benefits, even if enriched populations of specifically cytotoxic or cytostatic effectors are employed, and repeated administration of the cells would seem mandatory. The usual thresholds of safety for allogeneic white cell infusion may well be surpassed in the employment of such large inocula; and the patient's rejection responses are very likely to come into play in the course of prolonged, massive immunotherapy and to neutralize potential activity by the implanted effectors. The margins of security with regard to GvH disease excitation are also likely to be exceeded by the intensive immunotherapy with allogeneic cells that may have to be envisaged as requisite in man.

In theory, the problems of host-versus-graft and graft-versus-host reactions may not be beyond solution. Where the patient's own neoplastic cells are available for in vitro stimulation, close histocompatibility matching between patient and responder cell donor might lessen the eventualities of GvH disease and of accelerated rejection of the therapeutic graft. Moreover, techniques of proven efficacy have been developed in mice for selective immunoadsorption of clones reactive against normal allograft markers [48, 89]; in principle, there is no reason to believe that these are not applicable to human lymphoid cells, but the accompanying logistic problems may be difficult to surmount. Selective extirpation of effector cells with cytotoxic capacity against histocompatibility and other self-determinants could also be attempted by induced suicide with highly labeled thymidine, or with BUDR and light, upon exposure to the corresponding normal tissue antigens [12, 246]; such reduction in the numbers of anti-self clones, and use of allogeneic responder preparations representing some of the major self-determinants of the patient to be treated, may mitigate development of GvH reactivity appreciably. On the other hand, exposure of effector cells to radiation and certain chemicals risks the causation of new neoplastic transformations and of activation of latent virus. A safer procedure may lie with the induction in vitro of (partial) specific tolerance to normal tissue antigens of stimulating or target tumor cells [362]. Attempts in this direction may become more realistic with the advancing characterization of cell surface antigenic structure [108].

Work here in progress suggests that antihistocompatibility sensitization in culture can also be reduced by introduction into MLTC systems of antisera specific for the relevant markers, and by employment of antigen preparations subjected to treatments which inactivate the immunogenicity of (some) normal epitopes. Resort to medical management of GvH pathogenesis and symptomology may further attenuate the problem to moderate proportions. Findings in mice also suggest that permanent chimerism and chronic GvH pathology effected by allogeneic cells in immunosuppressed subjects might be prevented, without sacrifice of therapeutic goals, by administration of recipient-type hemopoietic and blood tissue [50]. Some control of premature rejection by the patient of allogeneic effector implants may be facilitated by circumspect chemical immunosuppression; and both GvH and host-versus-graft events might be circumscribable by the recently reported instrumentality of fractionated total lymphoid tissue irradiation [349].

Still other possibilities present themselves, along lines of histocompatibility apposition of responder, stimulator, and target, cells [133]. On the assumption of some TAA cross-reactivity between related neoplasms, it might be possible, for instance, to sensitize allogeneic responder cells against tumor stimulator cells derived from one patient, and to employ the effector clones produced in another. In that event, responder and stimulator cells should perhaps be as proximate as possible in histocompatibility makeup, so as to limit the generation of cytotoxicity against normal cell components. In contradistinction, the HL-A types of stimulator cells and of the patient to be treated should be distant, to lessen the likelihood of GvH phenomena due to whatever sensitization does occur against shared normal self-determinants. If multiple responder cell donors are required for an adequate supply of the therapeutic cells, it may be given to resort sequentially to responder cells from donors far removed from each other in HL-A characteristics, so as to minimize accelerated immunological rejection of each effector implant. Even then, the principle could be retained of restriction in overlap of strong histocompatibility antigens between the tumor stimulator cells in vitro and the tumor cells to be attacked in the patient, and of proximity between stimulator and responder cells; each new sensitization would then be with stimulator–responder combinations close in HL-A type, while preserving the distance of each individual combination from the others and from the patient to be treated.

Established lines of tumor cells seem less attractive for the purpose of MLTC stimulation, because of their antigenic and other instabilities, and because of their susceptibility to uncontrolled microbial contamination; nonetheless, their employment would solve logistic problems, and should not be ruled out at first sight.

Attention must also be given to avoidance of host rejection responses against implanted effector cells that might be caused by reactions directed at antigenic substances absorbed from the culture medium.

The translation of such schemes into reality will be a demanding task, technically and logistically as well as fundamentally. An immediate impediment to attempts at cross-sensitization may lie with the restriction imposed on cell-mediated immunological responses, especially against weak immunogens, by histocompatibility locus products. (It is noted, however, that MHC restriction of cell-mediated immune reactions to TAAs may not be as prevalent or decisive a limitation as was thought when the phenomenon was first described [170, 369]). A question to be explored is whether any such restriction could be sidestepped by sequential exposure of macrophages and T cells to the stimulating tumor cells or TAA preparations in culture, thereby invoking special helper effects toward the generation of cytotoxicity [385, 388]. Another basic conundrum lies with the functionality of cryopreserved effector cells. It has not yet been established that human effectors, or for that matter human neoplastic cells to be employed as stimulators, do in fact retain all required functional properties after prolonged storage at low temperatures; it is evident that some techniques of cryopreservation, storage, and thawing may impinge negatively on cell characteristics of immunological significance [22, 130]. Vital-dye exclusion and other standard laboratory tests for cell "viability" provide but dubious criteria of the ability of cells to discharge normal differentiated behavior upon implantation in a living host. The findings with murine stimulator and effector cells cryopreserved for a few weeks or months are encouraging, but they are not necessarily translatable to human cells, which may also have to be kept for much longer periods. It should be noted, on the other hand, that if cryopreservation proves successful for human material, it might have the added advantage of selective exclusion of suppressor clones, which in some experimental systems appear considerably less resistant to the procedure than cytotoxic effector and memory cells [269].

The normalcy of homing behavior of in vitro sensitized effector cells must also be questioned [383]. It has been observed, for instance, that such cells rapidly localize in the liver of syngeneic recipients following systemic introduction [60, 204], a decidedly aberrant deportment. Thus, even where effector cells are viable and functionally reactive after sensitization, cryopreservation, and thawing, their altered patterns of tissue localization – reflecting perhaps a degree of damage or alteration of the cells, or their absorption of culture constituents – may cause them to be rapidly sequestered and inactivated in vivo and to fail at reaching their intended targets. Further study is in order to determine whether any such problem can be solved, perhaps by recourse to small lymphocyte memory cells instead of reactive effector blasts.

Translatability of findings made in mouse models to the human clinical situation also appears problematic when the time dimension of therapeutic intervention is taken into account. The murine tumors against which passive/adoptive immunotherapy has proven felicitous (in combination with chemotherapy) kill their hosts within 3–4 weeks, very unlike the usual natural history of neoplastic disease in man. Even if cryopreserved human effectors should prove to retain full viability and normal performance upon administration to the patient, it remains questionable whether they can home in on residual tumor foci in sufficient numbers, and for the necessary time span, to carry out their intended activities before succumbing or suffering functional neutralization. In this regard, too, countermeasures can be conceived, but without any assurance at this time that the conceptions are realistic. One possibility to be explored is the direct introduction of effector cells into vessels afferent to large tumor deposits. Another, to facilitate ingress of the largest possible numbers of effector cells to solid tumor foci, lies with the possible elicitation of Shwartzman-like reactions in situ, or the employment of tumor necrotizing factor; disencumbered passage of cells from terminal blood vessels into the tumor mass or, as suggested by Vaage and Gandbhir [398], into the periphery of the nidus, may be a primary condition of efficacious intervention.

A major extrication from the difficulties of passive/adoptive cellular immunotherapy would be accomplished if it were possible to isolate the subcellular informational or recruitment principles [2, 5, 9, 103, 181, 295, 413] that may be responsible for the heightened resistance, and for the magnified sensitizability and effector capacity of responder cells, of subjects previously given allogeneic or syngeneic effector cells. If such entities could be substituted for intact cytotoxic effectors, the uncertainties and risks that becloud the application of whole, living cells would be obviated; this might also be true for irradiated or otherwise inactivated whole immune effector cells [2]. (It must be stressed that these uncertainties pertain not only to cell functionality in vivo, but that there is no information available as yet for human effector cells on any correlation between cytotoxic efficacy against tumor targets in vitro and therapeutic action in vivo. It is true that unfractionated, whole effector cell populations of mice evince such correlation, but evidence is also accruing in our experimental systems that distinct subpopulations of cells may be responsible for the in vitro and for the therapeutic effects, and it may be that the criterion of chromium liberation and similar short-term in vitro assays will offer faulty predictions of the usefulness of human effector cells.)

In summary, immunological intervention in neoplastic diseases of man is an exceedingly complicated task of "bioengineering" [280], requiring a sophisticated apprehension of immunological function and of host–tumor interactions still far beyond our reach. Neither has there been adduced so far a credible substructure of empirical information from truly pertinent animal tumor models to serve as reliable guidelines for clinical trial. Findings made in experimental systems may not, indeed, provide direct and detailed formulas for the clinician — there is always a quantum gap between laboratory and clinic — but they can help appreciably in indicating the latitudes of clinical investigation within which clinical answers must be sought; experimental models cannot be expected to yield solutions to problems of human medicine, but they are a required stepping-stone toward intelligent, focused clinical inquiry. It is in this light that the approach of passive/adoptive immunotherapy with effector cells generated in tissue culture takes on persuasiveness. Certainly, only clinical testing will tell what benefits can eventually be offered to the patients by this modality, and the step into the clinic will have to be taken with a large measure of cautious empiricism for all the encouragement that has already come and may continue to accrue from animal experiments. It is already evident, however, that the attempt at passive/adoptive immunotherapy with in vitro sensitized cells (and perhaps also with antibodies) is based on sound rationale, evades at least some of the formidable difficulties of active intervention in vivo, and can be categorically successful in animals. Most importantly, perhaps, the insights that will be obtained in the course of such ongoing laboratory and clinical investigation into the nature and kinetics of defensive immunological reactions against cancer and leukemia may open still further avenues of treatment, even if the strategy now pursued should fail as such to afford large therapeutic solutions.

4 Concluding Remarks

4.1 Immune Surveillance and Immunological Intervention: Hypothesis and Empiricism

The centrality of immunological mechanisms in the protection of species against progressive neoplastic disease is seriously questioned today. The theory of immunological surveillance derived its initial moment from observations made in a restricted range of experimental models, the relevance of which to clinical neoplasia has come under strong attack. Subsequent study of host–tumor relationships in human cancer and in spontaneously arising malignancies of laboratory animals has failed to confirm the generality of the theory's cornerstones: naturally appearing neoplastic cells do not always, or even commonly, express tumor-associated immunogenicity; where such immunogenicity is apparent, it is not regularly evocative of protective immune responses; progressive disease is not of necessity preceded or accompanied by prevalent immunological dyscrasia; putative escape modalities of neoplastic variants from immunological supervision cannot always be incriminated convincingly as the causes of advancing disease; and, in some circumstances, immunological reactions directed at neoplastic cells can exert protective and even stimulatory, rather than damaging, effects.

Various arguments are nonetheless still being marshalled in defense of the theory by some of its original proponents, and it may be true that those neoplastic processes that are seen in nature represent the rare exceptions to an indeed highly effective immunological surveillance. There is little doubt, however, that erosion of the theory's acceptance as the inclusive and pivotal statement of antitumor defense has undermined much of the enthusiasm for immunotherapy as a new and highly promising approach to the control of cancer.

A major purpose of this volume has been to suggest that authenticity of the hypothesis in its broad formulation is not a primary condition for efforts at clinical immunotherapy. The theory may be of cardinal interest to a comprehensive biological perspective of progressive neoplasia; it is not an indispensable framework for immunological intervention in cancer. Even if the current rearguard exercises at salvaging its orthodoxy fall short at convincing, there is a solid immunological basis for ongoing investment in the immunological approach to cancer treatment. The basis is provided by the considerable evidence for an at least minimal degree of antigenic distinction to neoplastic cells, by the recognized facility for translating low antigenicity and weak immunological responsiveness to levels sufficient for efficacious defensive reactivity, and by the opportunities for circumventing resistance impediments in the host by passive means of intervention. Support for this stance comes from consideration of the analogous circumstances of host–microbial parasite relationships, where efficacy of immunological measures, therapeutic and especially prophylactic, is demonstrable even against a background of inadequate responsiveness in the natural interaction. The fulcrum of our operative stance to tumor immunotherapy in the near future must be a pragmatic and empiric one, and extrication from the questionable fortunes of the theory of immunological surveillance seems a propitious step toward continued exploration.

4.2 Key Aspects of the Approaches to Tumor Immunotherapy

This essay outlines the likely avenues of investigation that present themselves toward the goal of effective immunotherapy in man. Each of the approaches weighed has both potential merit and inherent disadvantages, and each poses a set of similar and fundamental assignments. All demand, as a basic position by the investigator, the concurrence of a conservative empiricism in the clinic with concerted efforts to expand insight into the nature of immunological function and of the dynamics of host–tumor confrontation. Emphasis of consideration has been given to several specific tasks that seem insistent and immediate to the furthering of these efforts.

A methodology must be established for magnifying borderline antigenicity of TAAs to potent immunogenicity. The other side of the coin of this demand is the elaboration of knowledge of the functions and interactions of the diverse cellular, subcellular, and soluble elements which compose the immunological apparatus, and whose relative expression decides the quality and import of immunological responses. The final aim is elucidation of the genetic and environmental determinants which set the equilibria of immunological reactivity; the short-term commission is the pragmatic, quantitative definition of the activities of each phenotypic component, alone and in certain combinations, and under the impact of therapeutically intended manipulation.

An operative refocusing from the general to the particular is mandatory. It no longer seems possible to hazard inclusive propositions of the immunological and resistance capacities of species and strains. Rather, attention must center on the potentials for defense of the individual organism bearing a particular tumor; and, each therapeutic strategy must take cognizance of the variabilities that go with time and tissue locality of the neoplastic process and that are influenced by changes in the intrinsic and ambient environment of the host [146].

Recognition must be given in parallel to the selective pressures exerted on every neo-plastic cell population in every organism, and to the ensuing eventualities of selective and adaptive escape from host defenses. Correction or circumvention of both tumor avoidance and host inadequacy, genetic or circumstantial, thus becomes a key aspect of therapeutic planning.

Care to detail, even seemingly trivial, is requisite to every facet of immunological intervention. The large consequences that often accrue from minor variations in the pre-paration and application of immunotherapeutic reagents, active and passive, have been emphasized throughout this essay. A further, very recent example, may be mentioned: it is reported by Yarkoni and Rapp [446] that the concentration of oil in which several my-cobacterial moieties are suspended for intratumor injection has categorical effect on the ability of the substances to cause tumor regression and cure.

The obligation which devolves on the therapist from these considerations is more than formidable. Implied is the likelihood that immunotherapy may have to be tailored for each patient, and perhaps repeatedly in the course of disease. (Individual patient vagaries in responsiveness to immunomodulators is common clinical experience [185], paralleled by the variability of syngeneic mouse strains and of immunocytes taken from the animals to the immunopotentiating effects of MER, muramyl peptide, and other mi-crobial adjuvant moieties.) This condition seems fearsome and disappointing indeed if pondered in light of any early expectation that immunological treatment of cancer would prove to be a panacea attainable by simple and universal procedures. On reflection, however, the distance from other forms of therapy in neoplastic, and in many other, diseases is not as great as looms at first sight: more often than not, successful therapy, even with broadly active agents, is dependent on searching heed to the idiosyncracies of patient and disease.

In surveying the several major pathways of immunotherapy before us, deliberation has been given to the suggestive advantages of some. Such accent must be balanced, however, by clear acknowledgment of the large lacunae in the available information. No decision can be made today as to the immunological modality that will offer the greatest promise in a given type of disease. There is already persuasive experimental evidence, moreover, that maximum contributions of immunotherapy are often achieved only in conjunction with other forms of treatment. It now seems in order to explore as well the possibly additive or even synergistic efficacy of mixed immunological therapy. Both in the clinic and in the laboratory, immunotherapy of cancer has so far been limited largely to single-modality intervention. This may not be surprising in the early stages of a new approach; chemotherapy, too, was essayed at the outset largely as single-agent treatment, but the analogy should be extended: it has become obvious that multiple chemotherapeutic application is a generally far more effective means. Similarly, simul-taneous or sequential utilization of several immunotherapeutic methods, specific and nonspecific, active and passive, direct and auxiliary, would seem to hold the hope of an orchestrated punctuation of immunological responsiveness inhibitory to the tumor.

4.3 Goals and Expectations

What can be expected, realistically, of the contribution of immunotherapy to the total management of the cancer patient? Complete eradication of all neoplastic cells resident after conventional treatment is the obvious aspiration of all therapy. It does not appear probable, however, that immunological attack, even when coordinated with chemotherapy and radiation, can destroy every one of the large number of tumor cells often remaining in the tissues of patients even in full clinical remission. Total relief of the neoplastic burden by immunological measures seems a goal that will be reached only rarely, if ever.

On the other hand, even partial sterilization of neoplastic variants can tilt the balance of interaction in favor of the host. The natural history of neoplastic diseases suggests that the organism can often cope successfully and for prolonged periods of time with appreciable numbers of the pathogenic cells, by both immunological and nonimmunological mechanisms. Moreover, inhibition of the growth of neoplasms can be effected by immunological means, directly and by interference with tumor vascularization and with other tissue conditions requisite for unbridled neoplastic progression, even where tumor extinction is not afforded. A decisive slowing of tumor development is likely to be manifested by prolonged remission and survival, in itself no mean achievement today in the arena of malignant disease.

Immunological intervention could also alter the pathogenesis of neoplastic processes. It has been suggested, for instance, that various forms of immunotherapy may lead to an appreciable restriction in the extent of pulmonary metastasis of osteogenic sarcoma and other growths (61, 363; *H.S. Lawrence* 1977, personal communication, *H. Strander* 1979, personal communication), thereby perhaps affording new opportunities for surgical interference. The "peripheral" benefits of immunotherapy may also be not inconsiderable. Protection against life-threatening secondary infection can tide a patient through critical periods, and permit an intensity of chemo- and radiation therapy that would otherwise be forbidding. There is also the at least anecdotal impression in our experience with MER, and in that of other investigators with other immunotherapeutic agents, that pain, cachexia, and other symptoms of advancing disease may be ameliorated in some cases where the fatal course cannot be braked; improvement of only the quality of life of patients may be a limited achievement, but one that should not be dismissed.

4.4 Experimental Perspectives

That every clinical venture in tumor immunotherapy still stands in the shadow of large doubt is reflected by the repeated and obligatory resort in this paper to the conditional modals "may," "could," "might", and others. The field does not lend itself to certainty of statement. Its brief history has been beclouded by erratic swings of the pendulum to extremes of optimism and disappointment, neither founded on very solid grounds. What is badly wanted today is a constrained and balanced perspective and a great deal of solid work, both preparatory and applied.

The contributions of basic immunological science and of host–tumor relationship study are still too sparse to furnish firm, inclusive directions for rational clinical inquiry. It could be argued, perhaps, that want of knowledge also has its uses [143]. Firm assumption tends to channel exploration narrowly, toward confirmation of putative truths, and awareness in advance of all possible impasses can close experimental openings at incipience. It is often the unexpected "spin-off" from imaginative experimentation dared because no pretense of surety has curbed flair and adventure of plan, the lines of investigation seeming freer than indeed they may be, that holds the greatest reward (*G. Klein* 1978, personal communication).

A wide gap between laboratory and ward is invariable at best, moreover, and the more so where individual behavior in a biological system is marked by pervasive nonconformity. In the most auspicious circumstances, new clinical effort is guarded trial and error; in the area of tumor immunotherapy, it has been wildly speculative. The exigencies of the cancer problem do not justify a prolonged pause from any approach that holds out even remote hope, and clinical investigation will continue without awaiting development of a new corpus of fundamental insight. Nonetheless, every attempt must be made concurrently to speed the construction of relevant test systems of immunological and immune function, so that there can be a sustained and growing input into the clinical work of perception and judgment gathered at the bench. Too many of the stock-in-trade animal tumor models have been chosen for expedience, ease, productivity, and economy despite their obvious remove from anything resembling the nature and kinetics of spontaneous neoplasia. The dimensions of artificiality in cancer research, the distance between laboratory and clinic, need not be broadened unnecessarily.

It has been stressed elsewhere [425, 428] that a sine qua non to the construction of heuristic animal tumor models is the consideration that must be given to the totality of the relationship between tumor host and tumor cells. The intrinsic neoplastic potentials of transformed clones and the inherent resistance capacities of their host cannot in themselves explain susceptibility and resistance to neoplastic progression, any more than focus on potential parasite or on potential host alone can explain the vagaries of infectious disease evolution [92]. The web of host–parasite *interactions* represents and additional distinct, and critical dimension, set into the matrix of ambient environment of the interactants and of the intimate tissue environment in which each stage of the confrontation takes place. A case in point that has attracted much attention in recent years, and that may have large practical implications, is the multifaceted influence of diet on immunological reactivity and on resistance to cancer cells [100, 134, 135, 227]. Here, too, analogy to the host–parasite relationship in infectious diseases may be apt: Schneider demonstrated already several decades ago that certain dietary constituents can have a determinant effect on resistance to bacterial infection independent of any effects on the physiology of the animal and of the microbial organisms alone [324]. Full attainment of the ecological imperative is not given in experimental or clinical systems; neither is it allowable to refrain from every possible effort toward its approximation. It is never possible to control all the variables that impinge on a host–tumor relationship, but their existence must be acknowledged and must generate the awareness that all tumor processes are strikingly labile and fluctuating, increasingly so as they approach the natural circumstance. Only such cognizance can make for the modesty of interpretation of experimental results that is requisite for their realistic application to clinical study and trial.

It is not only artificiality of the supposed animal tumor analogs of human neoplasia that must be, and can be, contained. Preparatory study in man, and anecdotal and Phase I clinical investigation, also lend themselves to the greater intelligence of planning requisite for a plausible platform for wide immunotherapy trials. At least some of the many present lacunae in our ability to clear the way for definitive clinical study seem given to reduction by reasoned effort. A case in point that demands attention because it represents a major handicap to the advancement of tumor immunotherapy as art, if not for the time being as science, lies with the erratic association between immunological capacity as now assessed by various batteries of "immunological profile" testing and the level of resistance to neoplastic processes.

4.5 Immunological Capacity, Immunological Monitoring, and Susceptibility to Neoplastic Disease

Whereas some assays of "immune status" are in some cases seemingly revelatory of tumor risk following exposure to carcinogens [365], of the kinetics of resistance in the course of tumor growth [87, 157], and of the likely efficacy of immunotherapy [243], others are not, even in the same model and the same tumor host [87, 338A, 365]. In many other instances, no available yardstick of immunological strength has provided correspondent indications of the trend of malignant diseases [157, 403]. The deficiency in reliable correlates pertains to single animals and groups of syngeneic subjects as well as to the individual patient, and to resistance capacity both before and after immunological intervention. Nonspecific immunomodulators indeed often elevate some of the immunological functions assayed, and at times simultaneously heighten refractoriness to the disease process, but there is often little mutuality between the effects. This frequently holds true even where the immunological gauge measures reactivity in vitro or in vivo against TAAs, and where immunological treatment is with specific tumor vaccine preparations.

In the absence of guiding criteria, it is impossible to do precisely what appears mandatory for optimal immunotherapy: to adjust therapeutic modalities in light of fluctuating host responsiveness to challenging tumor cells and to extrinsic immunological stimulation in the course of disease. When conjecture takes the place of individually adapted, fluid intervention, as has been largely the case so far, the physician must await unmistakable clinical change before he can know whether he is working in right directions; and new investigational agents may be abandoned prematurely as ineffective for inauspicious surmises in trial design. Development of quantitative immunological capacity assays of correlative significance with host defensive ability, and with potentiation of immune status by therapy, is a task of considerable urgency.

It would appear more promising to find such correlations with assays measuring reactivity against the challenging tumor cells themselves than with tests for responsiveness to wholly unrelated antigenic and mitogenic entities; current studies by Herberman et al. on natural killer cells and on macrophage-mediated cytotoxicity (*R. B. Herberman* 1979, personal communication) confirm the observations of other workers in this direction. Even then, solution of the problem may prove to be formidable. Some, although not all, investigators incline to the view that immunocytes sequestered within tumor foci may possess greater antitumor reactivity, specific and nonspecific, than similar cells derived from the same host systemically [151, 153, 169, 183, 221, 403, 406]; in addition to negative findings, moreover, evidence has been brought forward that in situ immunocytes can exert negative effects on resistance [47]. It is wholly unclear at this point to what extent differences in host resistance against individual, dispersed foci of the same tumor accrue from the distinctive nature of the local tissue environment, the variant cytotoxic capabilities of immunocytes accumulating at the site from the general body pool or from local lymphoid centers (whose differential resistance functions have been described in numerous experimental systems), and the dissimilar expression of target antigens and immunoresistance by the neoplastic cells making up each lesion. The assumption is in order, then, that major attention should be given to the source of immunologically competent cells, and perhaps also to that of antibodies, which are to serve as reliable indicators of immune resistance. It also appears probable that comprehensive "scales" of antitumor reactions must be employed to attain a perspective of defensive status [345] in light of the uncertainty that any one test is representative of those responses to those antigens that make for resistance [157]; and that such assessment will have to include probes in the intact host, perhaps by procedures akin to the skin-window technique described by Black [41, 42] and Black et al. [43]. Immune failure at containment of neoplastic cells, as well as immune success, may be highly focused, even clonal, and only comprehensive testing is likely to be revealing.

The difficulties attending development of guiding criteria of host immunity to a tumor are more basic, however, than the assembly of indicatory tests with relevant immunocytes and soluble factors. As has been emphasized by many investigators during the past several years, the earlier view of idiopathic and intentionally induced gross immunodeficiency as a prerequisite for advancing neoplastic disease is not, in fact, borne out by the available evidence [228, 366, 403]. Although various immunodeficiency syndromes are not infrequently accompanied or succeeded by clinical cancer, the causal contribution of the former is often difficult to prove, and causality may be in the other direction as well [178, 283]. Laboratory animals (nude mice are a commonly cited example) and patients with other diseases who survive for long periods of time with marked immunological malfunction do not necessarily fall subject to neoplastic pathology; on the other hand, many cancer patients maintain seemingly normal immunological function, even late in the disease evolution. Can there be any reasonable hope, then, of developing immunological guidelines to patient treatment in more than the isolated instance?

The search might not be fruitless from the outset, and it will be aided by clear distinction between separate components of the question of relationship between immunological function and neoplasia. The malignant diseases that arise in nature may indeed not reflect immunological abnormality of the host or immune-neutralization by the tumor, where the neoplastic cells do not express operative immunogenicity. Moreover, any immunological defects that might be contributory to the genesis of some cancers may be different from those that make for further susceptibility once frank disease has occurred. The host of a growing neoplasm is subject to different stimuli, specific and nonspecific, and both conducive and unfavorable to immunological resistance, than is the healthy individual at the moment of initial challenge by transformed-cell proliferation. There may, in fact, be not indirect immunological measurements of "innate susceptibility" to cancer, and if there are they may have to ascertain other immunological capacities than those involved in the fluctuations of established disease [163].

Nonetheless, whatever may turn out to be the applicability of immunological probes to the characterization of persons with heightened risks of future cancer, and to the assessment and prognosis of defense in patients, there remains independently the definite possibility of monitoring immunological *intervention*. Here, even assays of responsiveness to tumor-unrelated antigens and to mitogens could conceivably be indicative, if cautiously interpreted, of a generally modulated responsiveness that could include antitumor capacity as well. Tests aimed at detecting, after immunological intervention, reactivity against the challenging or related neoplastic cells are still more likely to be of value. They subsume the eventuality that underlies all attempts at immunotherapy, that intervention accomplishes the translation of minimal tumor antigenicity to active immunogenicity, or the elevation of host immunological capability above critical thresholds; and they can be designed to take into account differential functionality of immunocytes of diverse tissue origin and the possible peculiarities of the in situ tumor circumstance. The possibility could also be entertained of applying tests that measure the effects of immunostimulation to normal, high-risk populations. Even if the immunological apparatus has little role in the hindrance of most nascent neoplastic foci, detection of certain immunological idiosyncrasies could identify individuals most likely to benefit from prophylactic *potentiation* of those categories of immunological responses that, upon magnification, take on defensive potential sufficient to restrict any later neoplasia at its inception [424].

4.6 Immunological and Nonimmunological Resistance to Progressive Neoplasia

This volume has focused on immunological parameters of host–tumor interactions, and has emphasized modalities of intervention designed to improve, or to arouse, immunological mechanisms of antitumor defense. It must be stressed, however, that other forms of opposition, not based on such reactions, are operative in tumor resistance, and may indeed play a primary role [1, 7, 373, 414, 458]. Some of the same cells that participate in specific immunological reactions can also undergo nonspecific activation in tissues to tumor cytotoxicity, and their then nonspecific tumoristatic and tumoricidal activities may represent a "first line of surveillance" [1]. Neoplastic deportment of variant clones is a manifestation of impairment in growth control, and basic, nonimmunological mechanisms for correction of faulty homeostasis have undoubtedly evolved. Recent findings point to pivotal cellular and molecular determinants of differential growth behavior. Malignancy has been linked closely to a structural abnormality in a particular membrane glycoprotein [53]; fibronectins and perhaps other components of basal laminae [401] may have decisive functions in setting normal tissue architectural patterns, and in differentiating between malignant and nonmalignant neoplasia; stromal tissue cells have been held accountable for setting the patterns of normal growth and differentiation and for restricting the malignant deportment of niduses of transformed tissues, and the suggestion has been made that they might also function as natural killer cells [83, 107, 350, 459]. A variety of normal, nonimmunological tissue factors may be able to discourage tumor development, especially at certain stages of ontogeny [373, 458, 459], or to reverse the neoplastic properties of transformed cells [83, 317]. Nonimmunological prevention of progressive neoplastic growth, invasion, and metastasis may be adaptive and acquired as well as native; and it may be most correct biologically to view specific immunological mechanisms as auxiliary defense superimposed on, and triggering and amplifying, more fundamental, archetypic modalities that assure the integrity of the multicellular organism [380, 414]. Here, too, the analogy of host–parasite relationship dynamics in infectious diseases may be instructive.

Distinction between normal self on the one hand and altered self and the alien on the other appears to be a property manifest very early in evolution, resident in primordial phagocytic and other connective tissue cells, and involved not only or even primarily in defense, but also in the differentiation of the organism, fixation of tissue matrices, and in feeding and reproductive behavior. The functions of lymphoid cells and of any of their evolutionary precursors or analogs, in themselves and by their diverse products, may be in essence supplementary and auxiliary. In facilitating intimacies of attachment and association, and in modulating the properties of other tissue cells, classic immunological function may have to be seen as a phylogenetically superimposed proficiency, providing in essence more effective means to pristine ends rather than a novel dimension of unrelated functionality. The responses already apparent in invertebrates to foreign particulate substances, and especially to pathogenetic microorganisms [390], tubercle formation in higher species [306], and the mechanical constraints placed on some tumors in mammals [398] are in some respects remarkably similar in their evolvement, cellular reactions seemingly representing the effector arms and humoral factors at times contributing to specificity of recognition and to the chemotactic mobilization of cellular elements. Lower animals and advanced species with a classic immunological apparatus display an essentially similar interdependence of cellular and humoral elements in the clearance of effete cells and in other physiological functions of immunological and immunological-like nature: antibodies and more primitive recognition molecules required to enlarge specificity of cell-mediated attack on unwanted and alien cells, various immunocytes necessary for antigen processing and the controlled production of recognition molecules.

It may not be apparent today how a more sophisticated perspective of the nature and weight of immunological reactivity will contribute to the design of better approaches to tumor immunotherapy, but it appears evident that the interaction between nonimmunological and immunological modes of resistance must be kept in view as constituting the totality of host immunity.

4.7 Coda

Lloyd Old has written recently that "the potential and power of immunological approaches to the cancer problem cannot be overemphasized, and it is difficult to think of an area of cancer research that is not benefitting from the application of immunological principles" [273]. Set in an appropriate biological perspective, this view may not be overoptimistic, for all the record of failure so far to accomplish great things by simplistic and even banal attempts in the realm of cancer immunotherapy. The efforts at decisive immunological intervention in neoplastic disease may turn out to be not wholly a labor of Sisyphus, if greater insight and imagination are brought to the task than a blind rolling of stones up steep inclines.

5 Notes added in Press

1. New evidence has recently been adduced by *Segal* et al. (*Segal, S., Siegal, T., Altaraz, H., Lev-El, A., Nevo, Z., Nebel, L., Katzenelson, A., Feldman,M.*: Fetal bone grafts do not elicit allograft rejection, due to protecting anti-Ia alloantibodies: Implication to the immune survival of fetuses in allogeneic mothers. Transpl., in press; *Segal, S.* Personal communications, 1979) for the possibility that certain fetal cells bear antigens of a molecular nature or arrangement making for the preferential evokation in the adult organism of immunological reponses that are not cytotoxic, and that may in fact facilitate the acceptance of foreign embryonic tissue grafts. The facilitation may be direct (enhancement mediated by certain molecular species of Ig), or indirect (inhibition of the synthesis or expression of other, cytotoxic elements). Animal and human females may be better capable of pro-

tective responsiveness against such determinants than males. Offered by these workers in possible explanation of maternal tolerance of the fetal homograft, the observations provide support for the premise of a qualitatively diverse immunogenicity by different categories of cellular antigen, singly or in conjunction with other cell surface constituents (which may come to expression progressively and variously as a function of time in development). The observations may also be of considerable significance for the understanding of escape mechanisms by tumor cells that express ontogenically pristine antigenic markers, and perhaps also of sex- and age-linked differences in the natural history of similar neoplastic diseases. The author expresses his appreciation of Prof. *Shraga Segal* of the Weizmann Institute for discussing this work, and its implications, with him.

2. The techniques of in vitro sensitization of anti-tumor effector cells, the nature of the antigens involved in stimmulator-responder/effector-target cell relationships and their genetic control and limits of restriction, and new experimental observations on passive/adoptive immunotherapy with cytotoxic lymphoid cells generated in culture are presented in greater detail in another, current review (*Kedar, E., Weiss, D.W.*: Cell-mediated tumor immunity induced in vitro. In: *Borek, F.,* (ed) Immunogenicity, 2nd ed., North-Holland Press, Amsterdam, in press).

3. A more detailed discussion of specificity and nonspecificity in biological interactions is presented in another, recent review article (*Weiss, D.W.*: Nonspecific immunity and cancer. In: *Kubica, G.P., Wayne, L.G.,* (eds) The Mycobacteria: A Sourcebook. Marcel Dekker Inc. New York to be published in 1980).

4. The possible role of mediators of humoral hypersensitivity – vasoamines – in tumor immunity, as well as in delayed-type hypersensitivity reactions to defined antigens, has been discussed recently by Askenase (Askenase, P.W. Role of basophils, mast cells, and vasoamines in hypersensitivity reactions with a delayed time course. Progr. Allergy *23*: 199–320, 1977).

Acknowledgements: The writer initiated work on this essay while Visiting Professor of Neoplastic Diseases in the laboratories of Professors *George Bekesi* and *James Holland* at Mt. Sinai Hospital and Medical School in New York, and wishes to express his gratitude to his hosts for their hospitality and for affording him the opportunity of the undertaking.
The help of a number of colleagues and friends is acknowledged with much appreciation: Drs. *Eli Kedar, Dov Sulitzeanu, David Naor, George Klein, Ron Herberman,* and *Eitan Yefenof* made many valuable and critical suggestions on the presentation and documentation of findings and ideas; Ms. *Gita Rubinstein* provided invaluable assistance as reference librarian; and Ms. *Belle Lerman* in the preparation of the manuscript. Mr. and Mrs. *Lawrence Tisch* warmly opened their home to the writer, who found there the opportunity and atmosphere conducive for writing (large sections of) the volume.

References

1.   *Alexander P* (1977): Innate host resistance to malignant cells not involving specific immunity. In: *Day SB, Myers WPL, Stansky P, Garattini S, Lewis MG* (eds). Cancer invasion and metastasis: biologic mechanisms and therapy. Raven, New York, pp 259–275

1A.   *Alexander P* (1976) Some immunologically based reactions that can cause regression of large tumor masses. Natl Cancer Inst Monogr 44:105–108

2.   *Alexander P, Delorme EJ* (1971) The use of irradiated immune lymphoid cells for immunotherapy of primary tumors in rats. In: *Weiss DW (ed)*. Immunological parameters of host-tumor relationships. Academic Press, New York, pp 239–245

3.   *Alexander P, Hall JG* (1970) The role of immunoblasts in host resistance and immunotherapy of primary sarcomata. Adv Cancer Res 13:1–37

4.   *Alexander P, Parr I* (to be published) BCG-induced resistance to tumors is caused by

selective recruitment of cytotoxic T-cells into sites of inflammation. In: *Spreafico F, Arnon R* (eds.) Tumor-associated antigens and their specific immune response. Academic Press, New York

5. *Alexander P, Delorme EJ, Hall JG* (1966) The effect of lymphoid cells from the lymph of specifically immunized sheep on the growth of primary sarcomata in rats. Lancet 1:1186–1189

5A. *Anderson PN, Klein DL, Bias WB, Mullins GM, Burke PJ, Santos GW* (1974) Cell-mediated immunological reactivity of patients and siblings to blast cells from adult acute leukemias. In: *Weiss DW (ed)* Immunological parameters of host-tumor relationships, vol III. Academic Press, New York, pp 219–237

6. *Anglin JH, Lerner MP, Nordquist RE* (1977). Blood group-like activity released by human mammary carcinoma cells in culture. Nature 269:254–255

7. *Apffel CA* (1976) Nonimmunological host defenses: a review. Cancer Res 36:1527–1537

8. *Arnon R* (to be published) Antitumor antibodies as carriers for anticancer drugs. In: *Spreafico F, Arnon R* (eds) Tumor-associated antigens and their specific immune response. Academic Press, New York

9. *Ascher MS, Gottlieb AA, Kirkpatrick CH* (eds) (1976) Transfer factor. Basic properties and clinical applications. Academic Press, New York

9A. *Asherson GL, Mayhew B* (1976) Induction of cell-mediated immunity in the mouse: circumstantial evidence for highly immunogenic antigen in the regional lymph nodes following skin painting with contact sensitizing antigens. In: *Weiss DW (ed)* Immunological parameters of host-tumor relationships, vol IV. Academic Press, New York, pp 174–187

10. *Attia MAM, Weiss DW* (1966) Immunology of spontaneous mammary carcinomas in mice. V. Acquired tumor resistance and enhancement in strain A mice infected with mammary tumor virus. Cancer Res 26:1787–1800

11. *Audibert F, Chedid L, Lefrancier P, Choay J* (1976) Distinctive adjuvanticity of synthetic analogs of mycobacterial water-soluble components. Cell Immunol 21:243–249

12. *Bach ML, Bach FH, Zoschke DC* (1973) Manipulation of immunologically reactive cell populations in vitro. Outline of an appoach to specific immunotherapy of cancer. In: *Weiss DW (ed)* Immunological parameters of host-tumor relationships, vol II. Academic Press, New York, pp 140–145

13. *Baker MA, Falk JA, Taub RN* (1978) Immunotherapy of human acute leukemia: antibody response to leukemia-associated antigens. Blood 52:469–480

14. *Baker PE, Gillis S, Smith KA* (1979) Monoclonal cytolytic T-cell lines. J Exp Med 149:273–278

15. *Baldwin RW* (1973) Immunological aspects of chemical carcinogenesis. Adv Cancer Res 18:1–75

15A. *Baldwin RW, Embleton MJ* (1969) Immunology of spontaneously arising rat mammary adenocarcinomas. Int J Cancer 4:430–439

16. *Baldwin RW, Embleton MJ* (1969) Immunology of 2-acetylaminofluorene induced rat mammary adenocarcinomas. Int J Cancer 4:47–53

17. *Baldwin RW, Pimm MV* (1978) BCG in tumor immuntherapy. Adv Cancer Res 28:91–147

18. *Baldwin RW, Price MR* (1975) Neoantigen expression in chemical carinogenesis. In: *Becker FF (ed)* Cancer. A comprehensive treatise, vol 1. Plenum Press, New York, pp 353–383

19. *Baldwin RW, Price MR* (1976) Immunobiology of rat neoplasia. Ann NY Acad Sci 276:3–10

20. *Bansal SC, Sjögren HO* (1974) Antitumor immune response and its manipulation in a tumor-bearing host. In: *Weiss DW (ed)*. Immunological parameters of host-tumor relationships, vol III. Academic Press, New York, pp 125–157

21. *Barski G, Youn JK, Francois D LE, Belehradek J Jr* (1974) Evolution of specific cell-bound immunity in hosts bearing solid tumors as related to tumor growth and treatment. In: *Weiss DW (ed)* Immunological parameters of host-tumor relationships, vol III. Academic Press, New York, pp 99–110

22. *Bartlett GL, Katsilas DC, Kreider JW, Purnell DM* (1977) Imunogenicity of "viable" tumor cells after storage in liquid nitrogen. Cancer Immunol Immunother 2:127–133

23. *Bauer H* (1974) Virion and tumor cell antigens of C-type RNA tumor viruses. Adv Cancer Res 20:275–341

24. *Bekesi JG, Holland JF* (1977) Active immunotherapy in leukemia with neuraminidase-modified leukemic cells. Recent Results Cancer Res 62:78–89

25. *Bekesi JG, Holland JF, Cuttner J, Silver R, Coleman M, Jarowski C, Vinceguerra V* (1976)

Immunotherapy in acute myelocytic leukemia (AML) with neuraminidase (n' ase) treated allogeneic myeloblasts with or without MER. Proc Am Assoc Cancer Res 17:184

26.   *Bekierkunst A* (1976) Immunotherapy of cancer with nonliving mycobacteria and chord factor (trehalose-6, 6'-dimycolate) in aqueous medium. J Natl Cancer Inst 57:963-964

27.   *Ben-Efraim S* (1977) Methanol extraction residue: effects and mechanisms of action. Pharmacol Ther [A] 1:383-410

28.   *Ben-Efraim S, Diamantstein T* (1975) Mitogenic and adjuvant activity of a methanol extraction residue (MER) of tubercle bacilli on mouse lymphoid cells in vitro. Immunol Commun 4:565-577

29.   *Ben-Efraim S, Weiss DW* (to be published) Effects of MER on lymphoid cell division and antibody synthesis in vitro. Cell Immunol

30.   *Ben-Efraim S, Constantini-Sourojon M, Weiss DW* (1973) Potentiation and modulation of the immune response of guinea pigs to poorly immunogenic protein-hapten conjugates by pretreatment with the MER fraction of attenuated tubercle bacilli. Cell Immunol 7:370-379

31.   *Ben-Efraim S, Teitelbaum R, Ophir R, Kleinman R, Weiss DW* (1974) Nonspecific modulation of immunological responsiveness in guinea pigs and mice by the tumor protective MER mycobacterial fraction: influence of condition of MER treatment and specific immunization, and effect of MER on early stages of the immune response. In: *Weiss DW (ed)* Immunological parameters of host-tumor relationships, vol III. Academic Press, New York, pp 158-169

32.   *Ben-Efraim S, Ulmer A, Schmidt M, Diamantstein T* (1976) Differences between lymphoid cell populations of guinea pigs and mice as determined by the response to mitogens in vitro. Int Arch Allergy Appl Immunol 51:117-130

33.   *Ben-Efraim S, Sarir C, Dar O, Barbash G, Weiss DW* (to be published) Effects of the MER tubercle bacillus fraction on the production of antibodies in vitro. I. Effect on the primary response. Cell Immunol

34.   *Ben-Sasson Z, Weiss DW, Doljanski F* (1974) Specific binding of factor(s) released by Rous sarcoma virus-transformed cells to splenocytes of chickens with Rous sarcomas. J Natl Cancer Inst 52:405-412

35.   *Bentwich Z, Weiss DW, Sulitzeanu D, Kedar E, Izak G, Cohen I, Eyal O* (1972) Antigenic changes on the surface of lymphocytes from patients with chronic lymphocytic leukemia. Cancer Res 32:1375-1383

36.   *Berrian JH, Brent L* (1958) Cell-bound antibodies in transplantation immunity. Ann NY Acad Sci 73:654-662

37.   *Bevan MJ, Cohn M* (1975) Cytotoxic effects of antigen- and mitogen induced T cells on various targets. J Immunol 114:559-565

38.   *Bevan MJ, Langman RE, Cohn M* (1976) H-2 antigen-specific cytotoxic T cells induced by concanavalin A: estimation of their relative frequency. Eur J Immunol 6:150-156

39.   *Billing R, Minowada J, Cline M, Clark B, Lee K* (1978) Acute lymphocytic leukemia-associated cell membrane antigen. J Natl Cancer Inst 61:423-429

40.   *Billington WD* (1969) Immunological processes in mammalian reproduction. In: *Adinolfi M, Humphrey J* (eds) Immunology and development. Heinemann Medical Books, London, pp 89-113

41.   *Black MM* (1972) Cellular and biologic manifestations of immunogenicity in precancerous mastopathy. Natl Cancer Inst Monogr 35:73-82

42.   *Black MM* (1973) Human breast cancer. A model for cancer immunology. In: *Weiss DW* (ed) Immunological parameters of host-tumor relationships, vol II. Academic Press, New York, pp 80-95

43.   *Black MM, Leis HP Jr* (1970) Human breast carcinoma. III. Cellular responses to autologous breast cancer: skin window procedure. NY State J Med 70:2583-2588

44.   *Blair PB* (1966) Immunology of the murine mammary-tumor virus (MTV): development of methods of assay. In: *Burdette WJ* (ed) Viruses inducing cancer. University Utah Press, Salt Lake City, pp 288-304

45.   *Blair PB* (1971) Immunological aspects of the relationship between host and oncogenic virus in the mouse mammary tumor system. In: *Weiss DW* (ed) Immunological parameters of host tumor relationships. Academic Press, New York, pp 161-186

46.   *Blair PB, Kripke ML, Lappé MA, Bonhag RS, Young L* (1971) Immunological deficiency

associated with mammary tumor virus (MTV) infection in mice: hemagglutinin response and allograft survival. J Immunol 106:364–370

47. *Blazar BA, Miller FR, Heppner GH* (1978) In situ lymphoid cells of mouse mammary tumors. III. In vitro stimulation of tumor cell survival by lymphoid cells separated from mammary tumors. J Immunol 120:1887–1891

48. *Bonavida B, Kedar E* (1974) Transplantation of allogeneic lymphoid cells specifically depleted of graft-versus-host reactive cells. Nature 249:658–659

49. *Bonnard GD, Schendel DJ, West WH, Alvarez JM, Maca RD, Yasaka K, Fine RL, Herberman RB, Landazuri MO De, Morgan DA* (to be published) Continued growth of normal human T lymphocytes in culture with retention of important functions. In: *Serrou B (ed)* Human lymphocyte differentiation. Its application to human cancer. Elsevier-North Holland Press, Amsterdam

50. *Boranic M* (1968) Transient graft-versus-host reaction in the treatment of leukemia in mice. J Natl Cancer Inst 41:421–437

51. *Bortin MM, Rimm AA, Rodey GE, Giller RH, Saltzstein EC* (1974) Prolonged survival in long passage AKR leukemia using chemotherapy, radiotherapy and adoptive immunotherapy. Cancer Res 34:1851–1856

52. *Bradley SG, Howe DB* (1976) Perturbation by bacterial lipopolysaccharide of the metabolic processes of human cells in continuous culture. J Reticuloendothel Soc 20:135–145

53. *Bramwell ME, Harris H* (1978) An abnormal membrane glycoprotein associated with malignancy in a wide range of different tumours. Proc R Soc Lond Biol 201:87–106

54. *Braun AC* (1975) Differentiation and dedifferentiation. In: *Becker FF* (ed) Cancer. A comprehensive treatise, vol 3. Plenum Press, New York, pp 3–20

55. *Brunda MJ, Minden P* (1977) Antibodies to bacterial and tumor-derived antigens in sera from normal guinea pigs. J Immunol 119:1374–1377

56. *Brunda MJ, Minden P, Heusser CH, Ferguson HR* (1978) Suppression of growth of guinea pig line 10 hepatocarcinoma. I. Effect of simultaneous administration of tumor cells and antibodies from normal rabbits. J Immunol 120:831–836

57. *Brunschwig A, Southam CM, Levin AG* (1965) Host resistance to cancer. Clinical experiments by homotransplants, autotransplants and admixture of autologous leucocytes. Ann Surg 162:416–425

58. *Burakoff SJ, Ratnofsky SE, Benacerraf B* (1977) Mouse cytolytic T lymphocytes induced by xenogeneic rat stimulator cells exhibit specificity for H-2 complex alloantigens. Proc Natl Acad Sci USA 74:4572–4576

59. *Burton DS, Blair PB, Weiss DW* (1969) Protection against mammary tumors in mice by immunization with purified mammary tumor virus (MTV) preparations. Cancer Res 29:971–973

60. *Burton RC, Warner NL* (1977) In vitro induction of tumor specific immunity. IV. Specific adoptive immunotherapy with cytotoxic T cells induced in vitro to plasmacytoma antigens. Cancer Immunol Immunother 2:91–99

61. *Byers VS, Levin AS, LeCam L, Johnston JO, Hackett AJ* (1976) Discussion paper: tumor-specific transfer factor therapy in osteogenic sarcoma: a two-year study. Ann NY Acad Sci 277:621–627

62. *Callewaert DM, Lightbody JJ, Kaplan J, Jaroszewski J, Peterson WD Jr, Rosenberg JC* (1978) Cytotoxicity of human peripheral lymphocytes in cell-mediated lympholysis; antibody-dependent cell mediated lympholysis and natural cytotoxicity assays after mixed lymphocyte culture. J Immunol 121:81–85

63. *Cantor H, Boyse E* (1977) Regulation of the immune response by T-cell subclasses. Contemp Top Immunobiol 7:47–67

64. *Carbone G, Invernizzi G, Meschini A, Parmiani G* (1978) In vitro and in vivo expression of original and foreign H-2 antigens and of the tumor-associated transplantation antigen of a murine fibrosarcoma. Int J Cancer 21:85–93

65. *Carey TE, Takahashi T, Resnick LA, Oettgen HF, Old LJ* (1976) Cell surface antigens of human malignant melanoma: mixed hemadsorption assays for humoral immunity to cultured autologous melanoma cells. Proc Natl Acad Sci USA 73:3278–3282

66. *Carrel S, Delisle M-C, Mach J-P* (1977) Antibody-dependent cell mediated cytolysis of human colon carcinoma cells induced by specific antisera against carcinoembryonic antigen. Can-

cer Res 37:2644–2650

67. *Caspary EA, Field EJ* (1971) Specific lymphocyte sensitization in cancer: is there a common antigen in human malignant neoplasia? Br Med J 2:613–617

68. *Chauvenet PH, Smith RT* (1978) Relationship of tumor-specific transplantation antigens to the histocompatibility complex: dissociation of in vitro alloantigen expression and in vivo alloimmunity from tumor-specific transplantation antigen strength. Int J Cancer 22:79–90

69. *Chedid L* (to be puplished) Therapeutic potential of immunoregulating synthetic glycopeptides. In: *Sela M, Chagas C* (eds) The role of nonspecific immunity in the prevention and treatment of cancer. Elsevier-North Holland Press, Amsterdam

70. *Chedid L, Audibert F* (1977) Chemically defined bacterial products with immunopotentiating activity. J Infect Dis 136:S246–S251

71. *Chedid L, Audibert F* (1977) Activity in saline of chemically well defined non-toxic bacterial adjuvants. In: *Miescher PA* (ed) Immunopathology, VIIth International Symposium. Schwabe, Basel, pp 382–396

72. *Chedid L, Audibert F, Lefrancier P, Choay J, Lederer E* (1976) Modulation of the immune response by a synthetic adjuvant and analogs. Proc Natl Acad Sci USA 73:2472–2475

73. *Chedid L, Parant M, Parant F, Lefrancier P, Choay J, Lederer E* (1977) Enhancement of nonspecific immunity to Klebsiella pneumoniae infection by a synthetic immunoadjuvant (N-acetyl-muramyl-L-alanyl-D-isoglutamine) and several analogs. Proc Natl Acad Sci USA 74:2089–2093

74. *Chedid L, Audibert F, Johnson AG* (1978) Biological activities of muramyl dipeptide, a synthetic glycopeptide analogous to bacterial immunoregulating agents. Prog Allergy 25:63–105

75. *Cheever MA, Kempf RA, Fefer A* (1977) Tumor neutralization, immunotherapy, and chemoimmunotherapy of a Friend leukemia with cells secondarily sensitized in vitro. J Immunol 119:714–718

76. *Cikes M, Friberg S Jr, Klein G* (1973) Progressive loss of H-2 antigens with concomitant increase of cell-surface antigen(s) determined by Moloney leukemia virus in cultured murine lymphomas. J Natl Cancer Inst 50:347–362

76A. *Clark DA, Necheles TF, Nathanson L, Whitten D, Silverman E, Flowers A* (1974) Apparent HL-A 5 deficiency in human malignant melanoma. II. HL-A 5 masking activity in sera of patients with progressive disease. In: *Weiss DW* (ed) Immunological parameters of host-tumor relationships, voll III. Academic Press, New York, pp 22–32

77. *Coggin JH Jr, Anderson NG* (1974) Cancer, differentiation, and embryonic antigens: some central problems. Adv Cancer Res 19:105–165

78. *Cohen IR,* (1973) The recruitment of specific effector lymphocytes by antigen-reactive lymphocytes in cell-mediated autosensitization and allosensitization reactions. Cell Immunol 8:209–220

79. *Cohen IR, Livnat S* (1976) The cell-mediated immune response: interactions of initiator and recruited T lymphocytes. Transplant Rev 29:24–58

80. *Cohen IR, Wekerle H, Feldman M* (1974) The regulation of self-tolerance. Implications for immune surveillance against tumor cells. Isr J Med Sci 10:1024–1032

81. *Cohen D, Yron I, Haber M, Robinson E, Weiss DW* (1975) Effect of treatment with the MER tubercle bacilli fraction on the survival of mice carrying mammary tumor isografts: injection of MER at the tumor site or at a distal location. Br J Cancer 32:483–489

82. *Cohen D, Yron I, Grover NB, Weiss DW* (1976) Chemoimmunotherapy of syngeneic mouse mammary carcinomas employing methanol extraction residue. Ann NY Acad Sci 277:195–208

83. *Cooper M, Pinkus H* (1977) Intrauterine transplantation of rat basal cell carcinoma as a model for reconversion of malignant to benign growth. Cancer Res 37:2544–2552

84. *Cuttner J, Glidewell OJ, Holland JF* (1978) A controlled trial of chemoimmunotherapy in acute myelocytic leukemia (AML). Proc Am Soc Clin Oncol 19:333

85. *Davies DAL* (to be published) Comparison of specific and non-specific approaches to clinical cancer immunotherapy. In: *Selas M, Chagas C* (eds) The role of nonspecific immunity in the prevention and treatment of cancer. Elsevier-North Holland Press, Amsterdam

86. *Davies M, Stewart-Tull DES, Jackson DM* (1978) The binding of lipopolysaccharide from Echerichia coli to mammalian cell membranes and its effect on liposomes. Biochim Biophys Acta 508:260–276

87. *Dean JH, Cannon GB, Jerrels TR, McCoy JL, Herberman RB* (to be published) Sensitive measurement of immunocompetence and anti-tumor reactivity in lung cancer patients and possible mechanisms of immunosuppression

88. *DeLeo AB, Shiku H, Takahashi T, John M, Old LJ* (1977) Cell surface antigens of chemically induced sarcomas of the mouse. I. Murine leukemia virus-related antigens and allo-antigens on cultured fibroblasts and sarcoma cells: description of a unique antigen on BALB/c meth A sarcoma. J Exp Med 146:720-734

89. *Devens B, Naor D, Kedar E* (to be published) Immune response to weakly immunogenic virally induced tumors. IV. Dissociated recognition of H-2 and tumor associated antigens. Transplantation

90. *Dezfulian M, Lavrin DH, Shen A, Blair PB, Weiss DW* (1967) Immunology of spontaneous mammary carcinomas in mice. Studies on the nature of the protective antigens. In: Carcinogenesis: a broad critique. Williams & Wilkins, Baltimore, pp 365-388

91. *Dezfulian M, Zee T, DeOme KB, Blair PB, Weiss DW* (1968) Immunology of spontaneous mammary carcinomas in mice. VI. Role of the mammary tumor virus in the immunogenicity of spontaneous mammary carcinomas of BALB/c mice and in the responsiveness of the hosts. Cancer Res 28:1759-1772

91A. *Diggelen OP van, Shin S, Phillips DM* (1977) Reduction in cellular tumorigenicity after mycoplasma infection and elimination of mycoplasma from infected cultures by passage in nude mice. Cancer Res 37:2680-2687

92. *Dubos RJ* (1954) Biochemical determinants of microbial disease. Harvard University Press, Cambridge

93. *Evans R, Alexander P* (1972) Mechanisms of immunologically specific killing of tumor cells by macrophages. Nature 236:168-170

94. *Falk L, Wright J, Wolfe L, Deinhardt F* (1974) Herpesvirus ateles: transformation in vitro of marmoset splenic lymphocytes. Int J Cancer 14:244-251

95. *Falk L, Johnson D, Deinhardt F* (1978) Transformation of marmoset lymphocytes in vitro with Herpesvirus ateles. Int J Cancer 21:652-657

96. *Fefer A* (1973) Adoptive tumor immunotherapy in mice as an adjunct to whole-body X-irradiation and chemotherapy. A review. In: *Weiss DW* (ed) Immunological parameters of host-tumor relationships, vol II. Academic Press, New York, pp 146-161

97. *Fell HB, Dingle JT, Coombs RRA, Lachman PJ* (1968) The reversible "dedifferentiation" of embryonic skeletal tissues in culture in response to complement-sufficient antiserum. In: *Warren KB* (ed) Differentiation and immunology. Academic Press, New York, pp 49-68

98. *Fenyö EM, Peebles PT, Wahlström A, Klein E, Cochran AJ* (1973) Changes in cell surface properties during the in vivo growth of Moloney lymphoma. In: *Weiss DW* (ed) Immunological parameters of host-tumor relationships, vol II. Academic Press, New York, pp 35-46

99. *Ferguson RM, Schmidtke JR, Simmons RL* (1977) Immunotherapy of experimental animals. In: *Green I, Cohen S, McCluskey RT* (eds) Mechanisms of tumor immunity. Wiley, New York, pp 193-214

100. *Fernandes G, Yunis EJ, Good RA* (1976) Suppression of adenocarcinoma by the immunological consequences of calorie restriction. Nature 263:504-507

101. *Fidler IJ* (to be published) Recognition and destruction of target cells by tumoricidal macrophages. In: *Weiss DW* (ed) Immunological parameters of host-tumor relationships, vol V. Academic Press, New York

102. *Fidler IJ, Nicolson GL* (1978) Tumor cell and host properties affecting the implantation and survival of blood-borne metastatic variants of B16 melanoma. Isr J Med Sci 14:38-50

103. *Fink MA* (ed) (1976) Immune RNA in neoplasia. Academic Press, New York

104. *Fish F* (1978) The effect of soluble tumor extracts on anti-tumor immune response. PhD, Tel Aviv University

105. *Flannery GR, Chalmers PJ, Rolland JM, Nairn RC* (1973) Immune response to a syngeneic rat tumor: development of regional node lymphocyte anergy. Br J Cancer 28:118-122

105A. *Folkman J* (1974) Tumor angiogenesis. Adv Cancer Res 19:331-358

106. *Forman J* (1977) T cell-mediated cytotoxicity against trinitrophenyl-modified cells: effect of glutaraldehyde treatment on the immunogenicity and antigenicity of trinitrophenyl-modified cells. J Immunol 118:1755-1762

107. *Friedenstein AJ, Chailakhyan RK, Latsinik NV, Panasyuk AF, Keiliss-Borok IV* (1974) Stro-

68   David W. Weiss

mal cells responsible for transferring the microenvironment of the hemopoietic tissues. Transplantation 17:331–340

108.   *Fuks A, Kaufman JF, Orr HT, Parham P, Robb RR, Terhorst C, Strominger JL* (1977) Structural aspects of the products of the human major-histocompatibility complex. Transplant Proc 9:1685–1689

109.   *Galili N, Naor D, Åsjö B, Klein G* (1976) Induction of immune responsiveness in a genetically low-responsive tumor-host combination by chemical modification of the immunogen. Eur J Immunol 6:473–476

110.   *Galili N, Devens B, Naor D, Becker S, Klein E* (1978) Immune responses to weakly immunogenic virally induced tumors. I. Overcoming low responsiveness by priming mice with a syngeneic in vitro tumor line or allogeneic cross-reactive tumor. Eur J Immunol 8:17–22

111.   *Galili U, Galili N, Vánky F, Klein E* (1978) Natural species-restricted attachment of human and murine T lymphocytes to various cells. Proc Natl Acad Sci USA 75:2396–2400

112.   *Galili U, Rosenthal L, Galili N, Klein E* (to be published) Activated T cells in the synovial fluid of arthritic patients: characterization and comparison with in vitro activated human and murine T cells in cooperation with monocytes in cytotoxicity. J Immunol

113.   *Gallily R, Duchan Z, Weiss DW* (1977) Potentiation of mouse peritoneal macrophage antibacterial functions by treatment of the donor animal with the methanol extraction residue fraction of tubercle bacilli. Infect Immun 18:405–411

114.   *Gallily R, Stain E, Weiss DW* (1977) Potentiation of macrophage activities following incubation with factor(s) released from lymphocytes treated in vitro with MER. J Reticuloendothel Soc 22:64a

115.   *Gallily R, Stain E, Weiss DW* (to be published) Potentiation of macrophage activities by the MER fraction in vitro. J Reticuloendothel Soc

116.   *Garrett TJ, Takahashi T, Clarkson BD, Old LJ* (1977) Detection of antibody to autologous human leukemia cells by immune adherence assays. Proc Natl Acad Sci USA 74:4587–4590

117.   *Garrido F, Schirrmacher V, Festenstein H* (1977) Studies on H-2 specificities on mouse tumour cells by a new microradioassay. J Immunogenet 4:15–27

118.   *Gershon RK* (1974) Regulation of concomitant immunity. Activation of suppressor cells by tumor excision. In: *Weiss DW* (ed) Immunological parameters of host-tumor relationships, vol. III. Academic Press, New York, pp 198–209

119.   *Gershon RK* (1977) Suppressor T cell dysfunction as a possible cause for autoimmunity. In: *Talal N* (ed) Autoimmunity. Genetic, immunologic, virologic, and clinical aspects. Academic Press, New York, pp 171–181

120.   *Gery I, Waksman BH* (1972) Potentiation of the T-lymphocyte response to mitogens. II. The cellular source of the potentiating mediator(s). J Exp Med 136:143–155

121.   *Gery I, Baer A, Stupp Y, Weiss DW* (1974) Further studies on the effects of the methanol extraction residue fraction of tubercle bacilli on lymphoid cells and macrophages. In: *Weiss DW* (ed) Immunological parameters of host-tumor relationships, vol III. Academic Press, New York, pp 170–177

122.   *Ghose T, Blair AH* (1978) Antibody-linked cytotoxic agents in the treatment of cancer: current status and future prospects. J Natl Cancer Inst 61:657–676

123.   *Ghose T, Tai J, Guclu A, Norvell ST, Bodurtha A, Aquino J, MacDonald AS* (1976) Antibodies as carriers of radionuclides and cytotoxic drugs in the treatment and diagnosis of cancer. Ann NY Acad Sci 277:671–689

124.   *Ghose T, Guclu A, Tai J, Norvell ST, MacDonald AS* (1976) Active immunoprophylaxis and immunotherapy in two mouse lymphoma models. J Natl Cancer Inst 57:303–315

125.   *Ghose T, Guclu A, Tai J, Mammen M, Norvell ST* (1977) Immunoprophylaxis and immunotherapy of EL4 lymphoma. Eur J Cancer 13:925–934

126.   *Gillis S, Smith KA* (1977) Long term culture of tumor-specific cytotoxic T cells. Nature 268:154–156

127.   *Glaser M* (1978) Adjuvant-induced thymus-derived suppressor cells of cell-mediated tumor immunity. Nature 275:654–656

128.   *Globerson A* (1976) In vitro approach to development to immune reactivity. Curr Top Microbiol Immunol 75:1–43

129.   *Goldstein AL, Cohen GH, Thurman GB* (1977) Potential role for thymosin in the treatment of primary immunodeficiency diseases and cancer. In: *Chirigos MA* (ed) Control of neoplasia

by modulation of the immune system. Raven Press, New York, pp 241–253

130.   *Golub SH* (1976) Cryopreservation of human lymphocytes. In: *Bloom BR, David JR* (eds) In vitro methods in cell-mediated and tumor immunity. Academic Press, New York, pp 731–735

131.   *Golub SH, Morton DL* (1974) Sensitization of lymphocytes in vitro against human melanoma associated antigens. Nature 251:161–163

132.   *Golub SH, Svedmyr EAJ, Hewetson JF, Klein G, Singh S* (1972) Cellular reactions against Burkitt lymphoma cells. III. Effector cell activity of leukocytes stimulated in vitro with autochthonous cultured lymphoma cells. Int J Cancer 10:157–164

133.   *Good RA* (1977) Cellular engineering. Clin Bull 7:33–39

134.   *Good RA, Fernandes G, Yunis EJ, Cooper WC, Jose DC, Kramer TR, Hansen MA* (1976) Nutritional deficiency, immunologic function, and disease. Am J Pathol 84:599–614

135.   *Good RA, Jose DC, Cooper WC, Fernandes G, Kramer TR, Yunis EJ* (1977) Influence of nutrition on antibody production and cellular immune responses in man, rats, mice, and guinea pigs. In: *Suskind RM* (ed) Malnutrition and the immune response. Raven Press, New York, pp 169–183

136.   *Gorsky Y, Vánky F, Sulitzeanu D* (1976) Isolation from patients with breast cancer of antibodies specific for antigens associated with breast cancer and other malignant diseases. Proc Natl Acad Sci USA 73:2101–2105

137.   *Gorsky Y, Weiss I, Sulitzeanu D* (1977) Complexes of breast-cancer-associated antigen(s) and corresponding antibodies in pleural effusions from patients with breast cancer. Isr J Med Sci 13:844–847

138.   *Granatek CH, Hanna MG Jr, Hersh EM, Gutterman JU, Mavligit GM, Candler EL* (1976) Fetal antigens in human leukemia. Cancer Res 36:3464–3470

139.   *Greene MI, Dorf ME, Pierres M, Benacerraf B* (1977) Reduction of syngeneic tumor growth by an anti-I-J alloantiserum. Proc Natl Acad Sci USA 74: 5118–5121

140.   *Greene MI, Perry LL, Benacerraf B* (to be published) Cross reactivity of alloantigens and tumor antigens in vivo. Implication for polymorphism. Proc ICN-UCLA Symp.

141.   *Gullino PM* (1975) Extracellular compartments of solid tumors. In: *Becker FF* (ed) Cancer. A comprehensive treatise, vol 3. Plenum Press, New York, pp 327–354

142.   *Gutterman JU* (1977) Cancer systemic active immunotherapy today – prospects for tomorrow. Cancer Immunol Immunother 2:1–9

143.   *Gutterman JU* (1978) Prospects for the future of immunotherapy: the need for individualism. In: Immunotherapy of human cancer, The University of Texas System Cancer Center, M.D. Anderson Hospital and Tumor Institute. 22nd Annual Clinical Conference on Cancer. Raven Press, New York, pp 395–406

144.   *Habel K* (1963) Immunologic aspects of oncogenesis by polyoma virus. In: Conceptual advances in immunology and oncology. 16th Annual Symposium of Fundamental Cancer Research, University of Texas, M.D. Anderson Hospital and Tumor Institute. Harper & Row, New York, pp 486–502

145   *Haller O* (to be published) Natural killer cells to leukemia: in vitro and in vivo studies. In: *Spreafico F, Arnon R* (eds) Tumor-associated antigens and their specific immune response. Academic Press, New York

146.   *Hanna MG Jr, Nettesheim P, Richter CB, Tennant RW* (1973) The variable influence of host microflora and intercurrent infections on immunological competence and carcinogenesis. In: *Weiss DW* (ed) Immunological parameters of host-tumor relationships, vol II. Academic Press, New York, pp 25–34

147.   *Haran-Ghera N* (1971) Influence of host factors on leukemogenesis by the radiation leukemia virus. In: *Weiss DW* (ed) Immunological parameters of host-tumor relationships. Academic Press, New York, pp 17–25

148.   *Haran-Ghera N* (1978) Spontaneous and induced preleukemia cells in C57B1/6 mice: brief communication. J Natl Cancer Inst 60:707–710

149.   *Harris TN, Harris S* (1976) Discussion paper: effect of IgG_1 class alloantibody on retention of skin allografts and on tumor growth in the mouse. Ann NY Acad Sci 277:700–705

150.   *Hart IR, Fidler IJ, Hanna MG Jr, Cardy RH, Gutterman JU, Hersh EM* (1978) The effects of intravenous administration of methanol extraction residue (MER) of tubercle bacilli in the dog. Cancer Immunol Immunother 3:229–238

151. *Haskill JS, Yamamura Y, Radov L* (1975) Host responses within solid tumors: non-thymus-derived specific cytotoxic cells within a murine mammary adenocarcinoma. Int J Cancer 16: 798–809

152. *Haskill JS, Radov LA, Yamamura Y, Parthenais E, Korn JH, Ritter FL* (1976) Experimental solid tumors: the role of macrophages and lymphocytes as effector cells. J Reticuloendothel Soc 20:233–241

153. *Haskill JS, Yamamura Y, Radov L, Parthenais E* (1976) Discussion paper: are peripheral and in situ tumor immunity related? Ann NY Acad Sci 276:373–380

154. *Henney CS, Tracey DE, Wolfe SA* (to be published) BCG-induced natural killer cells: immunotherapeutic implications. In: *Weiss DW* (ed) Immunological parameters of host-tumor relationships, vol V. Academic Press, New York

155. *Heppner GH, Calabresi P* (1972) Suppression by cytosine arabinoside of serum-blocking factors of cell-mediated immunity to syngeneic transplants of mouse mammary tumors. J Natl Cancer Inst 48:1161–1167

156. *Herberman RB* (1973) Cellular immunity to human tumor-associated antigens. In: *Weiss DW* (ed) Immunological parameters of host-tumor relationships, vol II. Academic Press, New York, pp 96–103

157. *Herberman RB* (1974) Cell-mediated immunity to tumor cells. Adv Cancer Res 19:207–263

158. *Herberman RB* (1977) Existence of tumor immunity in man. In: *Green I, Cohen S, McCluskey RT* (eds) Mechanisms of tumor immunity. Wiley, New York, pp 175–191

159. *Herberman RB* (to be published) Cytotoxicity against tumors by NK and K cells. In: *Spreafico F, Arnon R* (eds) Tumor-associated antigens and their specific immune response, Academic Press, New York

160. *Herberman RB, Holden HT* (1978) Natural cell-mediated immunity. Adv Cancer Res 27:305–377

161. *Herbermann RB, Campbell DA Jr, Oldham RK, Bonnard GD, Ting C-C, Holden HT, Glaser M, Djeu J, Oehler R* (1976) Immunogenicity of tumor antigens. Ann NY Acad Sci 276:26–44

162. *Herberman RB, Nunn ME, Holden HT, Staal S, Djeu JY* (1977) Augmentation of natural cytotoxic reactivity of mouse lymphoid cells against syngeneic and allogeneic target cells. Int J Cancer 19:555–564

163. *Hersh EM, Gutterman JU, Mavligit GM, Mountain CW, McBride CM, Burgess MA, Lurie PM, Zelen M, Takita H, Vincent RG* (1976) Immunocompetence, immunodeficiency, and prognosis in cancer. Ann NY Acad Sci 276:386–406

164. *Hewitt HB* (1978) The choice of animal tumors for experimental studies of cancer therapy. Adv Cancer Res 27:149–200

165. *Hewitt HB, Blake ER, Walder AS* (1976) A critique of the evidence for active host defence against cancer, based on personal studies of 27 murine tumours of spontaneous origin. Br J Cancer 33:241–259

166. *Hibberd AD, Metcalf D* (1971) Proliferation of macrophage and granulocyte precursors in response to primary and transplanted tumors. In: *Weiss DW* (ed) Immunological parameters of host-tumor relationships, Academic Press, New York, pp 202–210

167. *Hilgers J, Daams JH, Bentvelzen P* (1971) The induction of precipitating antibodies to the mammary tumor virus in several inbred mouse strains. In: *Weiss DW* (ed) Immunological parameters of host-tumor relationships, Academic Press, New York, pp 154-160

168. *Hirsch MS* (1976) Interactions between lymphocytes and C-type oncornaviruses in mice. In: *Weiss DW* (ed) Immunological parameters of host-tumor relationships, vol IV. Academic Press, New York, pp 127–133

169. *Holden HT, Haskill JS, Kirchner H, Herberman RB* (1976) Two functionally distinct anti-tumor effector cells isolated from primary murine sarcoma virus-induced tumors. J Immunol 117:440–446

170. *Holden HT, Landolfo S, Herberman RB* (1977) T-cell-dependent reactivity against tumor-associated antigens on allogeneic target cells. Transplant Proc 9:1149–1152

171. *Holland JF, Bekesi JG, Cuttner J* (1978) Chemoimmunotherapy for acute myelocytic leukemia. In: Immunotherapy of human cancer. The University of Texas System Cancer Center, M.D. Anderson Hospital and Tumor Institute. 22nd Annual Clinical Conference on Cancer. Raven Press, New York, pp 237–244

172. *Hollinshead AC* (1978) Active-specific immunotherapy. In: Immunotherapy of human can-

cer. The University of Texas System Cancer Center, M.D. Anderson Hospital and Tumor Institute. 22nd Annual Clinical Conference on Cancer. Raven Press, New York, pp 213–233

173. *Huebner RJ* (1967) Non-virion neoantigens in cells infected with and transformed by viruses. In: *Harris RJC* (ed) Specific tumour antigens. Munksgaard, Copenhagen, pp 265–272

174. *Hurwitz E, Maron R, Bernstein A, Wilchek M, Sela M, Arnon R* (1978) The effect in vivo of chemotherapeutic drug-antibody conjugates in two murine experimental tumor systems. Int J Cancer 21:747–755

175. *Immunopotentiation* (1973) Ciba Foundation Symposium 18 (new series). Elsevier-North Holland Press, Amsterdam

176. *Immunotherapy of human cancer* (1978) The University of Texas System Cancer Center, M.D. Anderson Hospital and Tumor Institute. 22nd Annual Clinical Conference on Cancer. Raven Press, New York

177. *International Cancer Research Workshop* on In situ Expression of Anti-Tumor Immunity. Tel Aviv: Tel Aviv University, June 4–7, 1978, to be published

178. *International Conference on Immunobiology of Cancer* (1976) Part III. Influence of the tumor process on immune mechanisms. Ann NY Acad Sci 276:386–492

179. *International Conference on Immunotherapy of Cancer* (1976) Part III. Specific active immunotherapy (tumor vaccines) for cancer. Ann NY Acad Sci 277:305–491

180. *International Conference on Immunotherapy of Cancer* (1976) Part IV. Specific adoptive immunotherapy of cancer. Ann NY Acad Sci 277:492–544

181. *International Conference on Immunotherapy of Cancer* (1976) Part V. Instructional methods of immunotherapy. Ann NY Acad Sci 277:545–633

182. *International Conference on Immunotherapy of Cancer* (1976) Part VI. Specific immunotherapy (antibodies) for treatment of cancer. Ann NY Acad Sci 277:634–715

183. *Ioachim HL* (1976) The stromal reaction of tumors: an expression of immune surveillance. J Natl Cancer Inst 57:465–475

184. *Israel L, Edelstein R* (1978) In vivo and in vitro studies on nonspecific blocking factors of host origin in cancer patients. Role of plasma exchange as an immunotherapeutic modality. Isr J Med Sci 14:105–130

185. *Izak G, Stupp Y, Manny N, Zajicek G, Weiss DW* (1977) The immune response in acute myelocytic leukemia. Effect of the methanol extraction residue fraction of tubercle bacilli (MER) on T and B cell functions and their relation to the course of the disease. Isr J Med Sci 13:677–693

186. *Jessup JM, Riggs CW, Hanna MG Jr* (1977) Influence of preexisting tumor immunity on Bacillus Calmette-Guerin immunotherapy of guinea pigs with both regional and disseminated tumor. Cancer Res 37:2565–2573

187. *Johnson TS, Hudson JL, Feldman ME, Irvin GL* (1975) III: Immunoprophylaxis and cytotoxic effector cells against EL4 leukemia induced in syngeneic C57B1/6J mice by use of irradiated EL4 cells. J Natl Cancer Inst 55:561–567

188. *Joklik WK* (1964) The intracellular uncoating of poxvirus DNA. II. The molecular basis of the uncoating process. J Mol Biol 8:277–288

189. *Jollès P, Paraf A* (1973) Chemical and biological basis of adjuvants. Mol Biol Biochem Biophys 13:1–147

190. *Jondal M, Targan S* (1978) In vitro induction of cytotoxic effector cells with spontaneous killer cell specificity. J Exp Med 147:1621–1636

191. *Juillard GJF, Boyer PJJ* (1977) Intralymphatic immunization: current status. Eur J Cancer 13: 439–440

192. *Juillard GJF, Boyer PJJ, Yamashiro CH, Snow HD, Weisenburger TH, McCarthy T, Miller RJ* (1977) Regional intralymphatic infusion (ILI) of irradiated tumor cells with evidence of distant effects. Cancer 39:126–130

193. *Kahan M, Bergman-Goldman R, Saltoun R, Naor D* (1976) Studies on the immune response to fixed antigens. Preferential induction of helper function with heavily trinitrophenylated sheep erythrocytes, and glutaraldehyde-treated sheep erythrocytes. J Immunol 117:16–22

194. *Kall MA, Hellström I* (1975) Specific stimulatory and cytotoxic effects of lymphocytes sensitized in vitro to either alloantigen or tumor antigens. J Immunol 114:1083–1088

195. *Kamo I, Friedman H* (1977) Immunosuppression and the role of suppressive factors in cancer. Adv Cancer Res 25:271–321

72   David W. Weiss

196.   *Karande A, Yefenof E, Fenyö EM, Klein G* (to be published) Moloney lymphoma cells express
       a polyprotein containing the gag gene-coded p15 and the Moloney leukemia virus-induced
       cell surface antigen (MCSA)
197.   *Kedar E, Lupu T* (1978) In vitro induction of cell-mediated immunity to murine leukemia
       cells. IV. Amplification of the generation of cytotoxic lymphocytes by enzymatically
       and chemically modified stimulator leukemia cells. J. Immunol Methods 21:35–50
198.   *Kedar E, Schwartzbach, M* (1979) Further characterization of suppressor lymphocytes indu-
       ced by fetal calf serum in murine lymphoid cell cultures: comparison with in vitro genera-
       ted cytotoxic lymphocytes. Cell Immunol 43:326–340
199.   *Kedar E, Vánky F* (to be published) Effect of the MER tubercle bacillus fraction on the in
       vitro sensitization of autochthonous peripheral blood lymphocytes against neoplastic cells
       in man
200.   *Kedar E, Unger E, Galili N, Klein G, Åsjö B, Bonavida B, Naor D* (1976) Immunogenicity of
       tumor cells modified by trinitrobenzene sulfonic acid (TNBS). Prog Clin Biol Res 9:109–121
201.   *Kedar E, Unger E, Schwartzbach M* (1976) In vitro induction of cell mediated immunity to
       murine leukemia cells. I. Optimization of tissue culture conditions for the generation of cy-
       totoxic lymphocytes. J Immunol Methods 13:1–19
202.   *Kedar E, Schwartzbach M, Raanan Z, Hefetz S* (1977) In vitro induction of cell-mediated im-
       munity to murine leukemia cells. II. Cytotoxic activity in vitro and tumor-neutralizing capa-
       city in vivo of anti-leukemia cytotoxic lymphocytes generated in macrocultures. J Immunol
       Methods 16:39–58
203.   *Kedar E, Schwartzbach M, Raanan Z, Hefetz S* (1978) In vitro induction of cell-mediated im-
       munity to murine leukemia cells. V. Adoptive immunotherapy of leukemia in mice with
       lymphocytes sensitized in vitro to leukemia cells. Cancer Immunol Immunother 4:151–159
204.   *Kedar E, Raanan Z, Schwartzbach M* (1978) In vitro induction of cell mediated immunity to
       murine leukemia cells. VI. Adoptive immunotherapy in combination with chemotherapy of
       leukemia in mice using lymphocytes sensitized in vitro to leukemia cells. Cancer Immunol
       Immunother 4:161–169
205.   *Kedar E, Nahas F, Unger E, Weiss DW* (1978) In vitro induction of cell-mediated immunity to
       murine leukemia cells. III. Effect of the methanol extraction residue (MER) fraction of
       tubercle bacilli on the generation of anti-leukemia cytotoxic lymphocytes. J Natl Cancer Inst
       60:1097–1106
206.   *Kedar E, Lupu T, Schwartzbach M, Avraham Y* (1979) In vitro induction of cell-mediated im-
       munity to murine leukemia cells. VII. Methods for augmenting the induction and expres-
       sion of the cytotoxic response in vitro to syngeneic tumors. J Immunol Methods 26:157–171
207.   *Kedar E, Raanan Z, Kafka I, Holland JF, Bekesi GJ, Weiss DW* (1979) In vitro induction
       of cytotoxic effector cells against human neoplasms. I. Sensitization conditions and effect of
       cryopreservation on the induction and expression of cytotoxic responses to allogeneic leu-
       kemia cells. J Immunol Methods 28:303–319
208.   *Kedar E, Nahas F, Schwartzbach M, Unger E, Raanan Z, Hefetz S, Weiss DW* (to be published)
       Generation in vitro of cytotoxic effector cells against syngeneic and allogeneic mouse leuke-
       mias and lymphomas. In: *Spreafico F, Arnon R* (eds) Tumor-associated antigens and their
       specific immune response. Academic Press, New York
209.   *Kirchner H, Glaser M, Herberman RB* (1975) Suppression of cell mediated tumour immunity
       by Corynebacterium parvum. Nature 257:396–398
210.   *Klein G* (1966) Humoral and cell-mediated mechanisms for host defense in tumor immunity.
       In: *Burdette WJ* (ed) Viruses inducing cancer. University Utah Press, Salt Lake City, pp 323–
       349
211.   *Klein G* (1966) Tumor antigens. Ann Rev Microbiol 20:223–252
212.   *Klein E* (1972) Tumor immunology; escape mechanisms. Ann Instit Pasteur 122:593–602
213.   *Klein G* (1975) Immunological surveillance against neoplasia. Harvey Lect 69:71–102
214.   *Klein G* (1975) Factors that interfere with or prevent effective destruction of tumors via im-
       mune mechanisms. In: *Smith RT, Landy M* (eds) Immunobiology of the tumor-host rela-
       tionship. Academic Press, New York, pp 203–213
215.   *Klein G* (1975) Chairman's remarks, session IV: factors that interfere with or prevent effec-
       tive destruction of tumors via immune mechanisms. In: *Smith RT, Landy M* (eds) Immuno-
       biology of the tumor-host relationship. Academic Press, New York, pp 201–276

216. *Klein G* (1977) Tumor-associated antigens in H-2 hemizygous isoantigenic variants of a somatic cell hybrid, derived from the fusion of 3-methylcholanthrene-induced sarcoma and a mammary carcinoma. J Natl Cancer Inst 58:383–386

217. *Klein G, Klein E* (1977) Rejectability of virus-induced tumors and nonrejectability of spontaneous tumors – a lesson in contrasts. Isr J Med Sci 13:666–676

218. *Klein G, KLein E* (1977) Immune surveillance against virus-induced tumors and nonrejectability of spontaneous tumors: Contrasting consequences of host versus tumor evolution. Proc Natl Acad Sci USA 74:2121–2125

219. *Klein G, Sjögren HO, Klein E* (1963) Demonstration of host resistance against sarcomas induced by implantation of cellophane films in isologous (syngeneic) recipients. Cancer Res 23:84–92

220. *Klein G, Friberg S Jr, Wiener F, Harris H* (1973) Hybird cells derived from fusion of TA3-Ha ascites carcinoma with normal fibroblasts. I. Malignancy, karyotype, and formation of isoantigenic variants. J Natl Cancer Inst 50:1259–1268

221. *Klein E, Becker S, Svedmyr E, Jondal M, Vánky F* (1976) Tumor infiltrating lymphocytes. Ann NY Acad Sci 276:207–216

222. *Klein G, Ehlin B, Witz I* (to be published) Further studies on a polyoma tumor associated membrane antigen. Int J Cancer

223. *Kleist S von* (1976) The use of CEA (carcinoembryonic antigen) and other carcinofoetal antigens in human cancer. In: *Wybran J, Staquet MJ* (eds) Clinical tumor immunology. Pergamon Press, New York, pp 89–103

224. *Kobayashi H, Sendo F, Kaji H, Shirai T, Saito H, Takeichi N, Hosokawa M, Kodama T* (1970) Inhibition of transplanted rat tumors by immunization with identical tumor cells infected with Friend virus. J Natl Cancer Inst 44:11–19

225. *Kobayashi H, Kodama T, Gotohda E* (1977) Xenogenization of tumor cells. Sando Printing, Sapporo Japan

226. *Koldovsky P* (1974) Carcinoembryonic antigen. Recent Results Cancer Res 45:1–69

227. *Kollmorgen GM, Sansig WA, Fischer G, Cunningham DE, Longley RE, Lehman AA, King MM, McCay PB* (to be published) A possible role of MER in protection against DMBA-induced tumors in rats fed different fat diets

228. *Kripke ML, Borsos T* (1974) Immunosuppression and carcinogenesis. A review. In: *Weiss DW* (ed) Immunological parameters of host-tumor relationships, vol III. Academic Press, New York, pp 74–89

229. *Kripke ML, Fisher MS* (1976) Immunologic parameters of ultraviolet carcinogenesis. J Natl Cancer Inst 57:211–215

230. *Kvist S, Ostberg L, Persson H, Philipson L, Peterson PA* (1978) Molecular association between transplantation antigens and cell surface antigen in adenovirus-transformed cell line. Proc Natl Acad Sci USA 75:5674–5678

231. *Lappé MA* (1969) Tumor specific transplantation antigens: possible origin in pre-malignant lesions. Nature 223:82–84

232. *Lappé MA* (1971) Evidence for immunological surveillance during skin carcinogenesis. Inflammatory foci in immunologically competent mice. In: *Weiss DW* (ed) Immunological parameters of host-tumor relationships. Academic Press, New York, pp 52–65

233. *Lappé M, Schalk J* (1971) Necessity of the spleen for balanced secondary sex ratios following maternal immunization with male antigen. Transplantation 11:491–495

234. *Lavrin DH, Blair PB, Weiss DW* (1966) Immunology of spontaneous mammary carcinomas in mice. III. Immunogenicity of C3H preoplastic hyperplastic alveolar nodules in C3Hf hosts. Cancer Res 26:293–304

235. *Lavrin DH, Blair PB, Weiss DW* (1966) Immunology of spontaneous mammary carcinomas in mice. IV. Association of the mammary tumor virus with the immunogenicitiy of C3H nodules and tumors. Cancer Res 26:929–934

236. *Leclerc C, Löwy I, Chedid L* (1978) Influence of MDP and of some analogous synthetic glycopeptides on the in vitro mouse spleen cell viability and immune response to sheep erythrocytes. Cell Immunol 38:286–293

237. *Lee SK, Oliver RTD* (1978) Autologous leukemia-specific T-cell-mediated lymphocytotoxicity in patients with acute myelogenous leukemia. J Exp Med 147:912–922

238. *Lengerova A* (1972) The expression of normal histocompatibility antigens in tumor cells.

Adv Cancer Res 16:235–271

239.   *Leshem B, Naor D* (1978) Studies on the immune response to fixed antigens. III. Induction of helper function for antibody-dependent cellular cytotoxicity responses. J Immunol 121: 401–408

240.   *Leventhal BG, Konior GS* (1977) Immunologic treatment of neoplasms in man. In: *Green I, Cohen S, McCluskey RT* (eds) Mechanisms of tumor immunity. Wiley, New York, pp 215–249

241.   *Levine P* (1976) Illegitimate blood group antigens P$_1$, A, and MN (T) in malignancy – a possible therapeutic approach with anti-T$_j^a$, anti-A, and anti-T. Ann NY Acad Sci 277:428–435

242.   *Levy R, Dilley J* (1977) The in vitro antibody response to cell surface antigens. II. Monoclonal antibodies to human leukemia cells. J Immunol 119:394–400

243.   *Levy JG, Whitney RB, Smith AG, Panno L* (1974) The relationship of immune status to the efficacy of immunotherapy in preventing tumor recurrence in mice. Br J Cancer 30:289–296

244.   *Lewis MG, Hartman D, Jerry LM* (1976) Antibodies and anti-antibodies in human malignancy: an expression of deranged immune regulation. Ann NY Acad Sci 276:316–327

245.   *Lotem J, Sachs L* (1978) In vivo induction of normal differentiation in myeloid leukemia cells. Proc Natl Acad Sci USA 75:3781–3785

246.   *Lukic ML, Leskowitz S* (1975) Cell-mediated immunity against allogeneic tumor after in vitro depletion of histocompatibility reactive cells. Proc Soc Exp Biol Med 148:420–423

247.   *Mantovani A* (to be published) Rationalized approaches to cancer chemoimmunotherapy. In: *Spreafico F, Arnon R* (eds) Tumor-associated antigens and their specific immune response. Academic Press, New York

248.   *Markson Y, Doljansky F, Weiss DW* (1978) Effects of prophylactic treatment with the methanol extraction residue fraction of tubercle bacilli (MER) on the development of Rous sarcomas of chickens following challenge with the Rous sarcoma virus. Isr J Med Sci 14:51–59

249.   *Markson Y, Doljansky F, Weiss DW* (to be published) Therapeutic effects of the methanol extraction residue fraction of tubercle bacilli (MER) on established Rous sarcomas of chickens. Cancer Immunol Immunotherapy

250.   *Martin GS* (1970) Rous sarcoma virus: a function required for the maintenance of the transformed state. Nature 227:1021–1023

251.   *Martin WJ, Wunderlich JR, MacDonald J* (1973) Suppressed development of cytotoxic lymphoid cells in tumor-immunized mice. In: *Weiss DW* (ed) Immunological parameters of host-tumor relationships, vol II. Academic Press, New York, pp 120–127

252.   *McKhann CF, Jagarlamoody SM* (1971) Evidence for immune reactivity against neoplasms. Transplant Rev 7:55–77

253.   *Medawar PB, Hunt R* (1978) Vulnerability of methylcholanthrene-induced tumours to immunity aroused by syngeneic foetal cells. Nature 271:164–165

254.   *Meidav A, Kedar E* (to be published) Properties of LAD, SD and CD determinants of normal and leukemic cells in mice. Isr J Med Sci

255.   *Melchers F, Potter M, Warner NL* (eds) (1978) Lymphocyte hybridomas. Curr Top Microbiol Immunol 81:

256.   *Mesa-Tejada R, Keydar I, Ramanarayanan M, Ohno T, Fenoglio C, Spiegelman S* (1978) Detection in human breast carinomas of an antigen immunologically related to a group-specific antigen of mouse mammary tumor virus. Proc Natl Acad Sci USA 75:1529–1533

257.   *Meschini A, Parmiani G* (1978) Anti-H-2 alloantibodies elicited by syngeneic immunizations with a chemically induced fibrosarcoma. Immunogenetics 6:117–123

258.   *Mihich E* (1969) Modification of tumor regression by immunologic means. Cancer Res 29: 2345–2350

259.   *Minden P, McClatchy JK, Wainberg M, Weiss DW* (1974) Shared antigens between Mycobacterium bovis (BCG) and neoplastic cells. J Natl Cancer Inst 53:1325–1331

260.   *Mitchell MS, Mokyr MB, Kahane I* (1975) Stimulation of lymphoid cells by components of BCG. J Natl Cancer Inst 55:1337–1343

261.   *Möller G, Möller E* (1962) Studies in vitro and in vivo of the cytotoxic and enhancing effect of humoral isoantibodies. Ann NY Acad Sci 99:504–530

262.   *Moertel CG, Ritts RE Jr, Schutt AJ, Hahn RG* (1975) Clinical studies of methanol extraction residue fraction of Bacillus Calmette-Guerin as an immunostimulant in patients with

advanced cancer. Cancer Res 35:3075–3083

263.   *Mokyr MB, Braun DP, Usher D, Reiter H, Dray S* (1978) The development of in vitro and in vivo anti-tumor cytotoxicity in noncytotoxic, MOPC-315-tumor-bearer, spleen cells "educated" in vitro with MOPC-315 tumor cells. Cancer Immunol Immunother 4:143–150

264.   *More R, Yron I, Weiss DW* (1978) In vitro studies on splenocyte cytotoxicity against syngeneic mammary carcinomas of mice. I. Reactivity of splenocytes from mice bearing mammary tumors against the corresponding and against other neoplasms. Isr J Med Sci 14:146–161

265.   *Motta R* (1971) Passive immunotherapy of leukemia and other cancer. Adv Cancer Res 14: 161–179

266.   *Naor D* (to be published) Suppressor cells: permitters and promoters of malignancy. Adv Cancer Res

267.   *Naor D, Galili N* (1977) Immune response to chemically modified antigens. Prog Allergy 22: 107–146

268.   *Naor D, Kahan M* (1977) Studies on the immune response to fixed antigens. II. Optimal conditions for inducing and eliciting helper function by fixed antigens and the mechanism responsible for this effect. Is J Med Sci 13:561–576

269.   *Naor D, O'Toole C* (1977) Cryopreservation of immunological memory and other lymphoid cell functions. J Immunol Methods 16:361–370

270.   *Nauts HC* (1969) The apparently beneficial effects of bacterial infections on host resistance to cancer. Monogr. 8, New York Cancer Instit. Publ., New York

271.   *Nilsson A, Révész L, Stjernswärd J* (1965) Suppression of strontium-90-induced development of bone tumors by infection with Bacillus Calmette-Guerin (BCG). Radiat Res 26:378–382

272.   *Nordquist RE, Hill Anglin J, Lerner MP* (1977) Antibody-induced antigen redistribuion and shedding from human breast cancer cells. Science 197:366–367

273.   *Old LJ* (1977) A special message, Scientific Advisory Council, Cancer Research Institute, Inc., New York

274.   *Old LJ, Stockert E* (1977) Immunogenetics of cell surface antigens of mouse leukemia. Annu Rev Genet 11:127–160

275.   *Orsini F, Pavelic Z, Mihich E* (1977) Increased primary cell mediated immunity in culture subsequent to adriamycin or daunorubicin treatment of spleen donor mice. Cancer Res 37:1719–1726

276.   *Ozer HL, Jha KK* (1977) Malignancy and transformation expression in somatic cell hybrids and variants. Adv Cancer Res 25:53–93

277.   *Palmer WN Jr, Swanson TL, Moore GE, Hyde PM* (1976) Immunogenicity of tumors alkylated with cyclohexyl-, benzyl-, or 2,4-dinitrophenylmethacrylate. Ann NY Acad Sci 277:412–427

278.   *Paluch E, Ioachim HL* (1978) Lung carcinoma-reactive antibodies isolated from tumor tissues and pleural effusions of lung cancer patients. J Natl Cancer Inst 61:319–324

279.   *Papsidero ID, Harvey SR, Snyderman MC, Nemoto T, Valenzuela L, Chu TM* (1978) Characterization of immune complexes from the pleural effusion of a breast cancer patient. Int J Cancer 21:675–682

280.   *Parish CR* (1972) The relationship between humoral and cell-mediated immmunity. Transplant Rev 13:35–66

281.   *Penn I* (1974) Malignancies in recipients of organ transplants. In: *Beers RF Jr, Tilghman RC, Basset EG* (eds) The role of immunological factors in viral and oncogenic processes. Johns Hopkins University Press, Baltimore, pp 211–221

282.   *Penn I* (1974) Letter to editor. Transplantation 18:284–285

283.   *Penn I* (1977) Development of cancer as a complication of clinical transplantation. Transplant Proc 9:1121–1127

284.   *Perloff M, Holland JF* (to be published) Adjuvant chemotherapy. In: *Holland JF, Frei E III* (eds) Cancer medicine, 2nd edn. Lea & Febiger, Philadelphia

285.   *Perloff M, Holland JF, Lumb GJ, Bekesi JG* (1977) Effects of methanol extraction residue of Bacillus Calmette-Guerin in humans. Cancer Res 37:1191–1196

286.   *Plata F, Cerottini JC, Brunner KT* (1975) Primary and secondary in vitro generation of cytolytic T lymphocytes in murine sarcoma virus system. Eur J Immunol 5:227–233

287.   *Pliskin ME, Prehn RT* (1978) Are tumor-associated transplantation antigens of chemically induced sarcomas related to alien histocompatibility antigens? Transplantation 26:19–24

288.   *Pollack S* (1973) Specific "arming" of normal lymph node cells by sera from tumor-bearing

mice. Int J Cancer 11:138–142

289. *Prager MD, Baechtel FS* (1973) Methods for modification of cancer cells to enhance their anti-genicity. In: *Busch H* (ed) Methods in cancer research, vol IX. Academic Press, New York, pp 339–400

289A. *Prager MD, Granatek CH, Ludden CM* (1976) Syngeneic and allogeneic mouse lymphoma antisera: specificity, reaction with fetal antigen and protective capacity. In: *Weiss DW* (ed) Immunological parameters of host-tumor relationships, vol IV. Academic Press, New York, pp 45–53

290. *Prehn RT* (1963) The role of immune mechanisms in the biology of chemically and physi-cally induced tumors. In: Conceptual advances in immunology and oncology. 16th Annual Symposium on Fundamental Cancer Research, Univ. of Texas M.D. Anderson Hospital and Tumor Institute. Harper & Row, New York, pp 475–485

291. *Prehn RT* (1973) Destruction of tumor as an "innocent bystander" in an immune response specifically directed against nontumor antigens. In: *Weiss DW* (ed) Immunological parame-ters of host-tumor relationships, vol II. Academic Press, New York, pp 171–175

292. *Prehn RT* (1976) Tumor progression and homeostasis. Adv Cancer Res 23:203–236

293. *Prehn RT* (1977) Immunostimulation of the lymphodependent phase of neoplastic growth. J Natl Cancer Inst 59:1043–1049

294. *Prehn RT, Lappé MA* (1971) An immunostimulation theory of tumor development. Trans-plant Rev 7:26–54

295. *Preisler HD, Jacobs SK* (to be published) Sensitization in vitro to murine myeloblastic leu-kemic cells by xenogeneic immune RNA. J Natl Cancer Inst

296. *Price MR, Baldwin RW* (1977) Shedding of tumor cell surface antigens. Cell Surface Rev 3: 423–471

297. *Radov LA, Haskill JS, Korn JH* (1976) Host immune potentiation of drug responses to a mu-rine mammary adenocarcinoma. Int J Cancer 17:773–779

298. *Rapp HJ* (1973) A guinea pig model for tumor immunology. A summary. In: *Weiss DW* (ed) Immunological parameters of host-tumor relationships, vol II. Academic Press, New York, pp 162–170

299. *Rapp HJ* (1976) Immunotherapy of experimental cancer as a guide to the treatment of hu-man cancer. Ann NY Acad Sci 276:550–556

300. *Rauscher FJ, O'Connor TE* (1973) Virology. In: *Holland JF, Frei E* III (eds) Cancer medicine, Lea & Febiger, Philadelphia, pp 15–44

301. *Reif AE, Robinson CM, Smith PJ* (1976) Preparation and therapeutic potential of rabbit anti-sera with "directed" specificities for mouse leukemias. Ann NY Acad Sci 277:647–669

302. *Reinisch CL* (1978) Induction of immunoregulatory T cells by adjuvant. Isr J Med Sci 14:89–97

303. *Reinisch CL, Andrew SL, Schlossman SF* (1977) Suppressor cell regulation of immune res-ponse to tumors: abrogation by adult thymectomy. Proc Natl Acad Sci USA 74:2989–2992

304. *Ribi E, Milner K, Kelly MT, Granger D, Yamamoto K, McLaughlin CA, Brehmer W, Strain SM, Smith RF, Parker R* (1976) Structural requirements of microbial agents for immunotherapy of the guinea pig line-10 tumor. In: *Lamoureux G, Turcotte R, Portelance V* (eds) BCG in can-cer immunotherapy Grune & Stratton, New York, pp 51–61

305. *Ribi E, McLaughlin CA, Cantrell JL, Brehmer W, Azuma I, Yamamura Y, Strain SM, Hwang KM, Toubiana R* (1978) Immunotherapy for tumors with microbial constituents or their syn-thetic analogues. A review. In: Immunotherapy of human cancer. The University of Texas System Cancer Center, M.D. Anderson Hospital and Tumor Institute. 22nd Annual Clini-cal Conference on Cancer. Raven Press, New York, pp 131–154

306. *Rich AA* (1951) The pathogenesis of tuberculosis, 2nd edn. Thomas, Springfield, Illinois, chapt XVIII, pp 713–789

307. *Ristow S, McKhann CF* (1977) Tumor-associated antigens. In: *Green I, Cohen S, McCluskey RT* (eds) Mechanisms of tumor immunity. Wiley, New York, pp 109–145

308. *Roder JC, Kiessling R* (1978) Target-effector interaction in the natrual killer cell system. I. Co-variance and genetic control of cytolytic and target-cell-binding subpopulations in the mouse. Scand J Immunol 8:135–144

309. *Röllinghoff M, Wagner H* (1973) In vivo protection against murine plasma cell tumor growth by in vitro activated syngeneic lymphocytes. J Natl Cancer Inst 51:1317–1318

310. *Röllinghoff M, Starzinski-Powitz A, Pfizenmaier K, Wagner H* (1977) Cyclophosphamide-sensitive T lymphocytes suppress the in vivo generation of antigen-specific cytotoxic T lymphocytes. J Exp Med 145:455–459

311. *Rook GAW* (1975) The potentiating, mitogenic and inhibitory effects on lymphocytes in vitro of macrophages in the lymph nodes of mice "overloaded" with mycobacterial products. Clin Exp Immunol 21:163–172

312. *Rook GAW, Stewart-Tull DES* (1976) The dissociation of adjuvant properties of mycobacterial components from mitogenicity, and from the ability to induce the release of mediators from macrophages. Immunology 31:389–396

313. *Rosenberg SA, Terry WD* (1977) Passive immunotherapy of cancer in animals and man. Adv Cancer Res 25:323–388

314. *Rosenberg SA, Schwarz S, Spiess PJ* (1978) In vitro growth of murine T cells. II. Growth of in vitro sensitized cells cytotoxic for alloantigens. J Immunol 121:1951–1955

315. *Rosenstreich DL, Oppenheim JJ* (1976) The role of macrophages in the activation of T and B lymphocytes in vitro. In: *Nelson DS* (ed) Immunobiology of the macrophage. Academic Press, New York, pp 161–199

316. *Rouse BT, Wagner H, Harris AW* (1972) In vivo activity of in vitro immunized lymphocytes. I. Tumor allograft rejection mediated by in vitro activated mouse thymocytes. J Immunol 108:1353–1361

317. *Sachs L* (1978) Control of normal cell differentiation and the phenotypic reversion of malignancy in myeloid leukemia. Nature 274:535–539

318. *Saint CYR CD-V* (1974) Modulation of expression of virus-induced tumor antigens in vivo and in vitro. In: *Weiss DW* (ed) Immunological parameters of host-tumor relationships, vol III. Academic Press, New York, pp 12–21

319. *Savary CA, Lotzova E* (1978) Suppression of natural killer cell cytotoxicity by splenocytes from Corynebacterium parvum-injected, bone-marrow tolerant, and infant mice. J Immunol 120:239–243

320. *Schechter B* (to be published) Elimination of tumor-enhancing cells and its effect on anti-tumor cytotoxic response. In: *Spreafico F, Arnon R* (eds) Tumor-associated antigens and their specific immune response. Academic Press, New York

321. *Schechter B, Feldman M* (1977) Hydrocortisone affects tumor growth by eliminating precursors of suppressor cells. J Immunol 119:1563–1568

322. *Schechter B, Treves AJ, Feldman M* (1976) Specific cytotoxicity in vitro of lymphocytes sensitized in culture against tumor cells. J Natl Cancer Inst 56:975–979

323. *Schlager SI, Dray S* (1976) Complete regression of a guinea pig hepatocarcinoma by immunotherapy with "tumor-immune" RNA or antibody to fibrin fragment E. Isr J Med Sci 12:344–359

324. *Schneider HJ* (1951) Nutrition and resistance-susceptibility to infection. Am J Trop Med 31:174–182

325. *Schrader JW, Cunningham BA, Edelman GM* (1975) Functional interactions of viral and histocompatibility antigens at tumor cell surfaces. Proc Natl Acad Sci USA 72:5066–5070

326. *Schroit AJ, Pagano RE* (1978) Introduction of antigenic phospholipids into the plasma membrane of mammalian cells: organization and antibody-induced lipid redistribution. Proc Natl Acad Sci 75:5529–5533

327. *Schwab JH* (1975) Suppression of the immune response by microorganisms. Bacteriol Rev 39:121–143

328. *Seigler HF, Shingleton WW, Metzgar RS, Buckley CE, Bergoc PM, Miller DS, Fetter BF, Phaup MB* (1972) Non-specific and specific immunotherapy in patients with melanoma. Surgery 72:162–174

329. *Sharma BS* (1976) In vitro lymphocyte immunization to cultured human tumor cells: parameters for generation of cytotoxic lymphocytes. J Natl Cancer Inst 57:743–748

330. *Sharma B, Terasaki PI* (1974) Immunization of lymphocytes from cancer patients. J Natl Cancer Inst 52:1925–1926

331. *Sharma B, Terasaki PI* (1974) In vitro immunization to cultured human tumor cells. Cancer Res 34:115–118

332. *Sharma B, Tubergen DG, Minden P, Brunda MJ* (1977) In vitro immunisation against human tumour cells with bacterial extracts. Nature 267:845–847

333. *Sharma B, Brunda MJ, Minden P* (to be published) Generation of cytotoxic lymphocytes against human tumor cells in vitro by a variety of soluble microbial extracts. J Natl Cancer Inst

334. *Shearer GM, Schmitt-Verhulst A-M* (1977) Major histocompatibility complex restricted cell-mediated immunity. Adv Immunol 25:55–91

335. *Shellam CR, Knight RA, Mitchison NA, Gorczynski RM, Maoz A* (1976) The specificity of effector T cells activated by tumours induced by murine oncornaviruses. Transplant Rev 29:249–276

336. *Shiku H, Takahashi T, Oettgen HF, Old LJ* (1976) Cell surface antigens of human malignant melanoma. II. Serological typing with immune adherence assays and definition of two new surface antigens. J Exp Med 144:873–881

337. *Shiku H, Takahashi T, Resnick LA, Oettgen HF, Old LJ* (1977) Cell surface antigens of human malignant melanoma. III. Recognition of autoantibodies with unusual characteristics. J Exp Med 145:784–789

338. *Shustik C, Cohen IR, Schwartz RS, Latham-Griffin E, Waksal SD* (1976) T lymphocytes with promiscuous cytotoxicity. Nature 263:699–701

338A. *Simmler MC, Rameau G, Chou MJ, Mathé G* (1976) Monitoring of nonspecific cell-mediated immunity in cancer patients. I. Frequent dissociation between the responses of skin tests to recall antigens and in vitro lymphocyte transformation. In: *Weiss DW* (ed) Immunological parameters of host-tumor relationships, vol IV. Academic Press, New York, pp 192–198

339. *Simmons RL, Rios A* (1973) Comparative and combined effect of BCG and neuraminidase in experimental immunotherapy. Natl Cancer Inst Monogr 39:57–65

340. *Simmons RL, Rios A* (1974) Cell surface modification in the treatment of experimental cancer: neuraminidase or concanavalin A. Cancer 34:1541–1547

341. *Sindelar WF, Ketcham AS* (1976) Regression of cancer following surgery. Natl Cancer Inst Monogr 44:81–84

342. *Sinkovics JG* (1976) Immunology of tumors in experimental animals. In: *Harris JE, Sinkovics JG* (eds) The immunology of malignant disease, 2nd edn. Mosby, Saint Louis, pp 93–282

343. *Sinkovics JG, Harris JE* (1976) Immunology and immunotherapy of human tumors. In: *Sinkovics JG, Harris JE* (eds) The immunology of malignant disease, 2nd edn, Mosby, Saint Louis, pp 410–579

344. *Sinkovics JG, Tebbi K, Cabiness JR* (1973) Cytotoxicity of lymphocytes to established cultures of human tumors: evidence for specificity. Natl Cancer Inst Monogr 37:9–18

345. *Shullenberger CC* (1976) chemoimmunotherapy for three categories of solid tumors (sarcoma, melanoma, lymphoma): the problem of immunoresistant tumors. In: *Crispen RG* (ed) Neoplasm immunity: mechanisms. ITR Press, Chicago, pp 193–212

346. *Sinkovics JG, Plager C, Papadopoulos N, McMurtrey MJ, Romero JJ, Waldinger R, Romsdahl MM* (1978) Immunology and immunotherapy of human sarcomas. In: Immunotherapy of human cancer. The University of Texas System Cancer Center, M.D. Anderson Hospital and Tumor Institute. 22nd Annual Clinical Conference on Cancer. Raven Press, New York, pp 267–288

347. *Siskind GW, Christian CL, Litwin SD* (eds) (1975) Immune depression and cancer. Grune and Stratton, New York

348. *Sjögren HO, Hellström I, Bansal SC, Hellström KE* (1971) Suggestive evidence that the "blocking antibodies" of tumor bearing individuals may be antigen-antibody complexes. Proc Natl Acad Sci USA 68:1372–1375

349. *Slavin S, Reitz B, Bieber CP, Kaplan HS, Strober S* (1978) Transplantation tolerance in adult rats using total lymphoid irradiation: permanent survival of skin, heart and marrow allografts. J Exp Med 147:700–707

350. *Slemmer G* (1972) Host response to premalignant mammary tissues. Natl Cancer Inst Monogr 35:57–71

351. *Smith RT* (1975) Chairman's remarks, session I: Tumor antigen as the controlling element in the tumor-host relationship. In: *Smith RT, Landy M* (eds) Immunobiology of the host-tumor relationship. Academic Press, New York, pp 3–68

352. *Snyderman R, Mergenhagen SE* (1976) Chemotaxis of macrophages. In: *Nelson DS* (ed) Immunobiology of the macrophage. Academic Press, New York pp 323–348

353. *Sparks FC, Albert NE, Andreone PA, Breeding JH* (1977) Effect of Bacillus Calmette-Guerin

on immunosuppression from cyclophosphamide, methotrexate, and 5-fluorouracil. Cancer Res 37:2560–2564

354. *Spontaneous Regression of Cancer, Conference on.* (1976) *Lewison EF* (ed) Natl Cancer Inst Monogr 44

355. *Steele G, Pierce GE* (1974) Effects of cyclophosphamide on immunity against chemically-induced syngeneic murine sarcomas. Int J Cancer 13:572–578

356. *Steinitz M, Feigis M, Weiss DW* (1975) Studies on the physiological manifestations of cell mediated cytotoxicity. II. Inhibition of ^{3}H-thymidine incorporation by plasmacytoma cells exposed in vitro to sensitized splenocytes. Cell Immunol 17:181–191

357. *Steinitz M, Koskimies S, Klein G, Mäkelä O* (1978) Establishment of specific antibody producing human lines by antigen preselection and EBV-transformation. Curr Top Microbiol Immunol 81:156–163

358. *Stewart-Tull DES, Shimono T, Kotani S, Knights BA* (1976) Immunosuppressive effect in mycobacterial adjuvant emulsions of mineral oils containing low molecular weight hydrocarbons. Int Arch Allergy Appl Immunol 52:118–128

359. *Stewart-Tull DES, Davies M, Jackson DM* (1978) The binding of adjuvant-active mycobacterial peptidoglycolipids and glycopeptides to mammalian membranes and their effect on artificial lipid bilayers. Immunology 34:57–67

360. *Stjernswärd J, Douglas P* (1977) Immunosuppression and metastasis. In: *Day SB, Laird Myers WP, Stansly P, Garattini S, Lewis MG* (eds) Cancer invasion and metastasis: biologic mechanisms and therapy (progress in cancer research and therapy, vol 5). Raven Press, New York pp 319–331

361. *Stolfi RL, Fugmann RA, Stolfi LM, Martin DS* (1974) Synergism between host anti-tumor immunity and combined modality therapy against murine breast cancer. J Natl Cancer Inst 13:389–403

362. *Stollar BD, Borel Y* (1976)•Nucleoside specificity in the carrier IgG-dependent induction of tolerance. J Immunol 117:1308–1313

363. *Strander H* (to be published) The interferon system and its possible use in the treatment of neoplastic disease. In: *Sela M, Chagas C* (eds) The role of nonspecific immunity in the prevention and treatment of cancer. Elsevier-North Holland Press, Amsterdam

364. *Stupp Y, Saltoun R, Weiss DW* (1976) Prevention by the MER tubercle bacillus fraction of immunosuppression induced by cancer chemotherapeutic agents. I. Antibody response of mice treated with cyclophosphamide. Cancer Immunol Immunother 1:219–226

365. *Stutman O* (1973) Immunological aspects of resistance to the oncogenic effect of 3-methylcholanthrene in mice. In: *Weiss DW* (ed) Immunological parameters of host-tumor relationships, vol II. Academic Press, New York, pp 13–24

366. *Stutman O* (1975) Immunodepression and malignancy. Adv Cancer Res 22: 261–422

367. *Stutman O* (1976) Correlation of in vitro and in vivo studies of antigens relevant to the control of murine breast cancer. Cancer Res 36:739–747

368. *Stutman O* (1977) Immunodeficiency and cancer. In: *Green I, Cohen S, McCluskey RT* (eds) Mechanisms of tumor immunity. John Wiley & Sons, New York, pp 27–53

369. *Stutman O, Shen F-W* (1978) H-2 restriction and non-restriction of T-cell-mediated cytotoxicity mouse mammary tumour targets. Nature 276:181–182

370. *Sugarbaker EV, Thornthwaite J, Ketcham AS* (1977) Inhibitory effect of a primary tumor on metastasis. In: *Day SB, Laird Myers WP, Stansly P, Garattini S, Lewis MG* (eds) Cancer invasion and metastasis: biologic mechnisms and therapy (progress in cancer research and therapy, vol 5). Raven Press, New York, pp 227–240

371. *Sulitzeanu D, Klein G, Morecky S, Gorsky Y* (1976) Coexistence in human sera of a cell (membrane?) antigen and of autoantibodies directed against it. Tissue Antigens 7:129–144

372. *Svet-Moldavsky GJ, Hamburg VP* (1967) An approach to the immunological treatment of tumors by artificial heterogenization. In: *Harris RJC* (ed) Specific tumour antigens. Munksgaard, Copenhagen, pp 323–327

373. *Svet-Moldavsky GJ, Zinzar SN, Karmanova NV* (1976) Inhibition of tumor and fetal tissue growth in newborn recipients. Ann NY Acad Sci 276:328–342

374. *Symoens J* (1977) Levamisole, an antianergic chemotherapeutic agent: an overview. In: *Chirigos MA* (ed) Control of neoplasia by modulation of the immune system. Raven Press, New York, pp 1–24

375.   *Tagliabue A, Herberman RB, McCoy JL* (1978) Cellular immunity to mammary tumor virus in normal and tumor-bearing C3H/HeN mice. Cancer Res 38:2279–2284

376.   *Tagliabue A, Herberman RB, Arthur LO, McCoy JL* (1979) Cellular immunity to tumor-associated antigens of transplantable mammary tumors of C3H/HeN mice. Cancer Res 39:35–41

377.   *Terry WD* (to be published) Overview of adjuvants in the immunotherapy of cancer. In: *Sela M, Chagas C* (eds) The role of nonspecific immunity in the prevention and treatment of cancer. Elsevier-North Holland Press, Amsterdam

378.   *Terry WD, Windhorst D* (eds) (1978) Immunotherapy of cancer: present status of trials in man. Raven Press, New York

379.   *Thomas L* (1959) Discussion. In: *Lawrence HS* (ed) Cellular and humoral aspects of the hypersensitive states. Hoeber-Harper, New York, pp 529–532

380.   *Thomas L* (1976) Possible mechanisms in regression. Natl Cancer Inst Monogr 44:137–139

381.   *Thomas ED, Bryant JI, Buckner CD, Clift RA, Fefer A, Jonson FL, Neiman P, Ramberg RE, Storb R* (1972) Leukaemia transformation of engrafted human marrow cells in vivo. Lancet 1:1310–1313

382.   *Thompson RB, Mathé G* (1972) Adoptive immunotherapy in malignant disease. Transplant Rev 9:54–72

383.   *Ting C-C* (1978) Studies of the mechanisms for the induction of in vivo tumor immunity. II. Distribution and homing of cytotoxic effector and precursor cells. J Natl Cancer Inst 60:437–444

384.   *Ting C-C, Bonnard GD* (1976) Cell-mediated immunity to Friend virus-induced leukemia. IV. In vitro generation of primary and secondary cell-mediated cytotoxic responses. J Immunol 116:1419–1425

385.   *Treves AJ* (1978) In vitro induction of cell-mediated immunity against tumor cells by antigen-fed macrophages. Immunol Rev 40:206–226

386.   *Treves AJ, Cohen IR, Feldman M* (1975) Immunotherapy of lethal metastases by lymphocytes sensitized against tumor cells in vitro. J Natl Cancer Inst 54:777–780

387.   *Treves AJ, Feldman M, Kaplan HS* (1977) In vitro sensitization of human lymphocytes against histiocytic lymphoma cell lines. I. Primary sensitization of lymphocyte subpopulations. J Immunol 119:955–960

388.   *Treves AJ, Feldman M, Kaplan HS* (1977) Macrophage-mediated in vitro sensitization of T-lymphocytes. I. Detection of murine leukemia virus-associated antigens. J Natl Cancer Inst 58:1527–1530

389.   *Triplett EL* (1962) On the mechanism of immunologic self recognition. J Immunol 89:505–510

390.   *Unestam T, Weiss DW* (1970) The host-parasite relationship between freshwater crayfish and the crayfish disease fungus Aphanomyces astaci: responses to infection by a susceptible and a resistant species. J Gen Microbiol 60:77–90

391.   *Uriel J* (1975) Fetal characteristics of cancer. In: *Becker FF* (ed) Cancer. A comprehensive treatise, vol 3. Plenum Press, New York, pp. 21–55

392.   *Vaage J* (1968) Nonvirus-associated antigens in virus-induced mouse mammary tumors. Cancer Res 28:2477–2483

393.   *Vaage J* (1973) Concomitant immunity and specific desensitization in murine tumor hosts. In: *Weiss DW* (ed) Immunological parameters of host-tumor relationships, vol II. Academic Press, New York, pp 128–139

394.   *Vaage J* (1974) Circulating tumor antigens versus immune serum factors in depressed concomitant immunity. Cancer Res 34:2979–2983

395.   *Vaage J* (1976) Protective serum effects in tumor immunity. Isr J Med Sci 12:334–343

396.   *Vaage J* (1978) In vivo and in vitro lysis of mouse cancer cells by antimetastatic effectors in normal plasma. Cancer Immunol Immunother 4:257–261

397.   *Vaage J, Agarwal S* (1977) Serum therapy for radiation-induced impairment of immune resistance to metastasis. Cancer Res 37:3556–3560

398.   *Vaage J, Gandbhir L* (1978) Local cellular responses associated with dormancy and regression of a syngeneic C3H mammary carcinoma. Cancer Immunol Immunother 4:263–268

399.   *Vaage J, Weiss DW* (1969) Immunization against spontaneous and autografted mouse mammary carcinomas in the autochthonous C3H/Crgl mouse. Cancer Res 29:1920–1926

400.   *Vaage J, Kalinovsky T, Olson R* (1969) Antigenic differences among virus-induced mouse mammary tumors arising in the same C3H host. Cancer Res 29:1452-1456

401.   *Vaheri A, Ruoslahti E, Mosher DF* (eds) (1978) Fibroblast surface proteins. Ann NY Acad Sci 312:1-456

402.   *Vánky F, Klein E, Stjernswärd J, Nilsonne U, Rodriguez L, Péterffy Á* (1978) Human tumor – lymphocyte interaction in vitro. II. Conditions which improve the capacity of biopsy cells to stimulate autologous lymphocytes. Cancer Immunol Immunother 5:63-69

403.   *Vánky F, Klein E, Stjernswärd J, Rodriguez L, Péterffy Á, Steiner L, Nilsonne U* (1978) Human tumor-lymphocyte interaction in vitro. III. T lymphocytes in autologous tumor stimulation (ATS). Int J Cancer 22:679-686

404.   *Vogl SE, Lumb, G, Bekesi JG, Holland JF* (1977) Preclinical study of iv administration of the methanol extraction residue of Bacillus Calmette-Guerin. Cancer Treat Rep 61: 901-903

405.   *Vose BM, Vánky F, Fopp M, Klein E* (1978) In vitro generation of cytotoxicity against autologous human tumor biopsy cells. Int J Cancer 21:588-593

406.   *Vose BM, Vánky F, Klein E* (1977) Human tumour-lymphocyte interaction in vitro. V. Comparison of the reactivity of tumour-infiltrating, blood and lymph-node lymphocytes with autologous tumour cells. Int J Cancer 20:895-902

407.   *Wagner H, Feldman M, Boyle W, Schrader JW* (1972) Cell-mediated immune response in vitro. III. The requirement for macrophages in cytotoxic reactions against cell-bound and subcellular alloantigens. J Exp Med 136:331-343

408.   *Wainberg MA, Phillips ER* (1976) Immunity against avian sarcomas. A review. In: *Weiss DW* (ed) Immunological parameters of host-tumor relationships. vol IV. Academic Press, New York, pp 108-126

409.   *Wainberg MA, Markson Y, Weiss DW, Doljanski F* (1974) Cellular immunity against Rous sarcomas of chickens. Preferential reactivity against autochthonous target cells as determined by lymphocyte adherence and cytotoxicity tests in vitro. Proc Natl Acad Sci USA 71:3565-3569

410.   *Wainberg MA, Markson Y, Doljanski F, Weiss DW* (1975) Reactivity of serum from Rous-sarcoma-bearing chickens with autochthonous and with allogeneic tumor cells: preferential autochthonous recognition. Int J Cancer 15:985-994

411.   *Wainberg MA, Deutsch V, Weiss DW* (1976) Stimulation of anti-tumor immunity in guinea-pigs by methanol extraction residue of BCG. Br J Cancer 34:500-508

412.   *Wainberg MA, Margolese RG, Weiss DW* (1977) Differential responsiveness of various substrains of inbred strain 2 guinea pigs to immunotherapy with the methanol extraction residue (MER) of BCG. Cancer Immunol Immunother 2:101-108

413.   *Wang BS, Onikul SR, Mannick JA* (1978) Prevention of death from metastases by immune RNA therapy. Science 202:59-60

414.   *Ward PA, Cohen S* (1977) Regulation of inflammatory responses in neoplastic disease. In: *Green I, Cohen S, McCluskey RT* (eds) Mechanisms of tumor immunity. Wiley, New York, pp 305-313

415.   *Weiss DW* (1958) Inhibition of tuberculin skin hypersensitivity in guinea pigs by injection of tuberculin and intact tubercle bacilli during fetal life. J Exp Med 108:83-104

416.   *Weiss DW* (1967) Immunology of spntaneous tumors. In: *Lecam I, Neyman J* (eds) Proceedings of the fifth Berkeley symposium on mathematical statistic and probability, vol IV: biology and problems of health. University of Califonia Press, Berkeley, pp 657-706

417.   *Weiss DW* (1969) Immunological parameters of host-tumor relationships: spontaneous mammary neoplasia of the inbred mouse as a model. Cancer Res 29:2368-2373

418.   *Weiss DW* (1969) Immunological parameters of the host-parasite relationship in neoplasia. Ann NY Acad Sci 164:431-448

419.   *Weiss DW* (1972) Summary: antigens in preneoplastic tissue during tumorigenesis. Natl Cancer Inst Monogr 35:89-100

420.   *Weiss DW* (1972) Nonspecific stimulation and modulation of the immune response and of states of resistance by the MER fraction of tubercle bacilli. Natl Cancer Inst Monogr 35:157-171

421.   *Weiss DW* (1974) Immunological intervention in neoplasia. In: The role of immunological factors in viral and oncogenic processes. Johns Hopkins Med J [Suppl] 3:131-169

82 David W. Weiss

422. *Weiss DW* (1976) MER and other mycobacterial fractions in the immunotherapy of cancer. Med Clin North Am 60:473–497
423. *Weiss DW* (1976) Neoplastic disease and tumor immunology from the perspective of host-parasite relationships. Natl Cancer Inst Monogr 44:115–122
424. *Weiss DW* (1977) The questionable immunogenicity of certain neoplasms: what then the prospects for immunological intervention in malignant disease? Cancer Immunol Immunother 2:11–19
425. *Weiss DW* (1978) Animal models of cancer immunotherapy: some considerations. In: Immunotherapy of human cancer. The University of Texas System Cancer Center, M.D. Anderson Hospital and Tumor Institute. 22nd Annual Clinical Conference on Cancer. Raven Press, New York, pp 101–109
426. *Weiss DW* (1978) Discussions. In: *Terry WD, Windhorst D* (eds) Immunotherapy of cancer. Raven Press, New York
427. *Weiss DW* (1978) Host mechanisms for control of tumor growth that can be modulated by nonspecific immunotherapy. In: Immunotherapy of human cancer. The University of Texas System Cancer Center, M.D. Anderson Hopital and Tumor Institute. 22nd Annual Clinical Conference on Cancer. Raven Press, New York, pp 41–61
428. *Weiss DW* (to be published) Animal models of cancer immunotherapy: questions of relevance. Cancer Treat Rep
429. *Weiss DW* (to be published) Approaches to "nonspecific" immunotherapy of cancer with microbial immunomodulators. In: *Sela M, Chagas C* (eds) The role of nonspecific immunity in the prevention and treatment of cancer. Elsevier-North Holland Press, Amsterdam
430. *Weiss DW* (In press) Tumor immunology and immunotherapy in 1977. In: *Weiss DW* (ed) Immunological parameters of host-tumor relationships. Vol. 5 Academic Press, New York
431. *Weiss B, Sachs L* (1978) Indirect induction of differentiation in myeloid leukemic cells by lipid A. Proc Natl Acad Sci USA 75:1374–1378
432. *Weiss DW, Yashphe DJ* (1973) Nonspecific stimulation of antimicrobial and antitumor resistance and of immunological responsiveness by the MER fraction of tubercle bacilli. In: *Zuckerman A, Weiss DW* (eds) Dynamic aspects of host-parasite relationships. Academic Press, New York, pp 163–223
433. *Weiss DW, Bonhag RS, Parks JA,* (1964) Studies on the heterologous immunogenicity of a methanol-insoluble fraction of attenuated tubercle bacilli (BCG). I. Antimicrobial protection. J Exp Med 119:53–70
434. *Weiss DW, Faulkin LF Jr, DeOme KB* (1964) Acquisition of heightened resistance and susceptibility to spontaneous mouse mammary carcinomas in the original host. Cancer Res 24:732–741
435. *Weiss DW, Sulitzeanu A, Young L, Adelberg M, Segev Y* (1971) Studies on the immunogenicity of preneoplastic and neoplastic mammary tissues of BALB/c mice free of the mammary tumor virus. In: *Weiss DW* (ed) Immunological parameters of host-tumor relationships. Academic Press, New York, pp 187–201
436. *Weiss DW, Kuperman O, Fathallah N, Kedar E* (1976) Mode of action of mycobacterial fractions in anti-tumor immunity: preliminary evidence for a direct nonspecific stimulatory effect of MER on immunologically reactive cells. Ann NY Acad Sci 276:536–549
437. *Welsh RM* (1978) Opinion. Mouse natural killer cells: induction, specificity, and function. J Immunol 121:1631–1635
438. *West WH, Cannon GB, Kay HD, Bonnard GD, Herberman RB* (1977) Natural cytotoxic reactivity of human lymphocytes against a myeloid cell line: characterization of effector cells. J Immunol 118:355–361
439. *Westphal O* (to be published) Anti-tumor effects of bacterial endotoxin (lipopolysaccharides, lipid A) and synthetic lysolecithin analogues. In: *Sela M, Chagas C* (eds) The role of nonspecific immunity in the prevention and treatment of cancer. Elsevier-North Holland Press, Amsterdam
440. *White RG* (1968) Antigens and adjuvants. Proc R Soc Med 61:1–5
441. *Wilkinson PC* (1976) Cellular and molecular aspects of chemotaxis of macrophages and monocytes. In: *Nelson DS* (ed) Immunobiology of the macrophage. Academic Press, New York, pp 349–365

442.   *Witz IP* (1977) Tumor-bound immunoglobulins: in situ expressions of humoral immunity. Adv Cancer Res 25:95–148

443.   *Witz IP, Lee N, Klein G* (1976) Serologically detectable specific and cross-reactive antigens on the membrane of a polyoma virus-induced murine tumor. Int J Cancer 18:243–249

444.   *Woods MW, Landy M, Whitby JL, Burk D* (1961) Symposium on bacterial endotoxins. III. Metabolic effects of endotoxins on mammalian cells. Bacteriol Rev 25:447–456

445.   *Yagel S, Gallily R, Weiss DW* (1975) Effect of treatment with the MER fraction of tubercle bacilli on hydrolytic lysozomal enzyme activity of mouse peritoneal macrophages. Cell Immunol 19:381–386

446.   *Yarkoni E, Rapp HJ* (to be published) Influence of oil concentration on the efficacy of tumor regression by emulsified components of mycobacteria. Cancer Res

447.   *Yoffee J, Weiss DW* (to be published) Histological changes in the livers of inbred mice following intravenous injection of the MER tubercle bacillus fraction. Israel J Med Sci

448.   *Yoshida, T, Cohen S* (1977) Lymphokines in tumor immunity. In: *Green I, Cohen S, McCluskey RT* (eds) Mechanisms of tumor immunity. Wiley, New York, pp 87–108

449.   *Yron I, Cohen D, Robinson E, Haber M, Weiss DW* (1975) Effects of methanol extraction residue and therapeutic irradiation against established isografts and simulated local recurrence of mammary carcinomas. Cancer Res 35:1779–1790

450.   *Yron I, Cohen D, Grover N, Weiss DW* (to be published) Immune response toward a murine methylcholanthrene-induced sarcoma: comparison of in vivo and in vitro assays. Israel J Med Sci

451.   *Yu A, Watts H, Jaffe N, Parkman R* (1977) Concomitant presence of tumor-specific cytotoxic and inhibitor lymphocytes in patients with osteogenic sarcoma. New Eng J Med 298:121–127

452.   *Zarling JM, Raich PC, Mc Keough M, Bach FH* (1976) Generation of cytotoxic lymphocytes in vitro against autologous human leukaemia cells. Nature 262:691–693

453.   *Zarling JM, Robins HI, Raich PC, Bach FH, Bach ML* (1978) Generation of cytotoxic T lymphocytes to autologous human leukemia cells by sensitization to pooled allogeneic normal cells. Nature 274:269–270

454.   *Zimber C, Ben-Efraim S, Weiss DW* (1977) Prevention by the MER tubercle bacillus fraction of immunosuppression induced by cancer chemotherapeutic agents. II. Contact hypersensitivity in guinea pigs and mice treated with cyclophosphamide. Cancer Immunol Immunother 3:35–42

455.   *Zimber C, Ben-Efraim S, Weiss DW* (to be published) Prevention by the MER tubercle bacillus fraction of immunosuppression induced by cancer chemotherapeutic agents. III. Contact hypersensitivity in guinea pigs and mice treated with 5-fluorouracil and methotrexate. Cancer Immunol Immunotherapy

456.   *Zinkernagel RM* (1978) Speculation on the role of major transplantation antigens in cell-mediated immunity against intracellular parasites. Curr Top Microbiol Immunol 82:113–138

457.   *Zinkernagel RM, Doherty PC* (1975) H-2 compatibility requirement for T-cell-mediated lysis of target cells infected with lymphocytic choriomeningitis virus. Different cytotoxic T-cell specificities are associated with structures coded for in H-2K or H-2D. J Exp Med 141:1427–1436

458.   *Zinzar SN, Svet-Moldavsky GJ, Karmanova NV* (1976) Nonimmune and immune surveillance. I. Growth of tumors and normal fetal tissues grafted into newborn mice. J Natl Cancer Inst 57:47–55

459.   *Zinzar SN, Svet-Moldavsky GJ, Karmanova NV* (1978) Nonimmune and immune surveillance. II. The effect of the recipients' age, tumor immunogenicity and neonatal thymectomy on the phenomenon of tumor growth inhibition. J Natl Cancer Inst 61:737–745

460.   *Zöller M, Price MR, Baldwin RW* (1976) Inhibition of cell-mediated cytotoxicity to chemically induced rat tumours by soluble tumour and embryo cell extracts. Int J Cancer 17:129–137

Lymphocyte Hybridomas

Second Workshop on "Functional Properties of Tumors of T and B Lymphocytes". Sponsored by the National Cancer Institute (NIH) April 3–5, 1978 Bethesda, Maryland, USA

Editors: F. Melchers, M. Potter, N. Warner

Reprint. 1979. 85 figures, 86 tables. XXI, 246 pages
ISBN 3-540-09670-1

(Originally published as **Current Topics in Microbiology and Immunology, Volume 81**)

Plasma cell-plasmacytoma hybrids are a unique source of homogeneous antibodies with extraordinary specificity. Since the original discovery by Köhler and Milstein, many laboratories have become actively engaged in making lymphocyte hybrids of normal and malignant cells, mainly to produce homogeneous antibodies specific for a wide variety of interesting antigens. In addition, thes hybrids have become useful as models for studying T-cell functions and lymphocyte growth regulation and differentiation, as a means for studying the location of genes expressed in lymphocytes, immunoglobulins, and for the study of the biochemical basis of neoplastic change.

The second workshop on "Functional Properties of Tumors T and B Lymphocytes" was held in April 1978 at the National Institutes of Health, Bethesda, Maryland, USA, bringing together the world's leading experts in this field. This book publishes the proceedings of that workshop and represents an impressive summary of the scientific progress and the technical know-how of many laboratories working on lymphocyte fusions, a technique which is currently gaining wide interest in immunology, molecular and cellular biology, biochemistry and medical research.

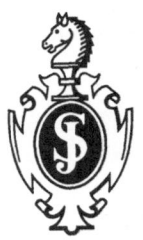
Springer-Verlag
Berlin
Heidelberg
New York

Other Volumes of Interest from this Series

Springer-Verlag
Berlin
Heidelberg
New York

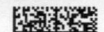